On the Death of a Child

On the Death of a Child

THIRD EDITION

CELIA HINDMARCH
BA (Hons)
MBACP Accredited Counsellor
MBACP Accredited Supervisor

Radcliffe Publishing
Oxford • New York

Radcliffe Publishing Ltd
18 Marcham Road
Abingdon
Oxon OX14 1AA
United Kingdom

www.radcliffe-oxford.com
Electronic catalogue and worldwide online ordering facility.

First edition 1993
Second edition 2000

Celia Hindmarch has asserted her right under the Copyright, Designs and Patents Act 1998 to be identified as the author of this work.

British Library Cataloguing in Publication Data

A catalogue record for this book is available from the British Library.

ISBN-13: 978 1 84619 403 0

Typeset by Pindar NZ, Auckland, New Zealand
Printed and bound by Cadmus Communications, USA

Contents

Preface

While the death of a child is a comparatively rare event in the Western world, it remains one of the greatest challenges to anyone supporting those affected by it.

Childhood is associated with hope, promise, innocence and joy, and the loss of a child is always emotive. Some high-profile child deaths, such as the murder of Rhys Jones in Liverpool and the abusive neglect of Baby P in Haringey, bring public outrage as well as private grief. Others, such as the death of Ivan Cameron, are inspirational as well as intensely sad, in this case challenging society's preconceptions of disability.

'Ivan's death was tragic. His life was not.'

This life-affirming statement by Ivan's father David, leader of the Conservative Party at the time of his son's death, echoes a new dimension which I have sought to bring to this third edition.

Essentially, the addition of **Chapter 10**, *Hope, meaning and resilience*, includes interviews with parents who reveal how the experience of losing a child can build resilience, derive meaning from their child's life, and inspire hope for the future. Elsewhere in the book the reader is challenged by the tragedy of the death: here the reality is balanced by hope. These parents have found purpose in fund-raising, public awareness, lobbying, and the development of new support resources, as legacies from their children.

This is in keeping with the original inspiration for this book which came from the first years of the Alder Centre, founded 20 years ago in 1989, and still going strong. The Alder Centre is situated at the Royal Liverpool Children's NHS Trust Hospital Alder Hey. Its remit is *to support all those affected by the death of a child*, of whatever age and from whatever cause. The Centre was initiated by a group of bereaved parents who recognised not only their own need for support but the potential for supporting others through their experience. Their vision drove a partnership with professionals to provide a multi-purpose resource centre that became a model for good practice nationally and internationally. Bereaved parents became keynote speakers at conferences for health professionals, developed a telephone helpline (now the Child Death helpline in conjunction with Great Ormond Street), organised support groups and family holidays.

The observations and guidelines offered here are thus grounded in practical experience. Basic learning has been gained by following the first guiding principle which is advocated for professionals offering support: *to listen to what individual people say they want rather than presuming what they need*. The only experts are bereaved family members themselves.

Chapter 10 reflects some new understandings of grief explored in **Chapter 2**, *Features of grief and mourning when a child dies*. I have been inspired by Yalom's notion of 'rippling' as a helpful way to derive meaning from a child's life, however limited. This can be particularly helpful for those who have no religious faith in life after death to give them comfort. Other new understandings of grief outlined in Chapter 2 include the evolution of ideas that build on traditional models. These fresh concepts move away from the medical treatment model and towards one that is characterised by growth, empowerment and the normalisation of grief.

Those familiar with earlier editions will also note the addition of further professional roles in **Chapter 3** – pathologists, bereavement support workers, mortuary technicians and coroners – to acknowledge their important contributions to the support of bereaved families.

This is a book to dip into rather than be read from cover to cover. It is limited by the experiences of most contributors coming from a predominantly white, Western cultural perspective. Against the background of ever-increasing publications on child death, this book remains distinctive in offering guidelines as a checklist against varying levels of experience. Ways of coping have to be found that avoid hard-nosed denial at one extreme and compassion fatigue at the other. From theory and narrative come practical ideas of how to be, what to say, what to do, how to look after yourself, and how to stay humble. Hopefully this book will give you reassurance that, whatever contact you have with the family, and however inadequate you may feel, you *can* make a difference.

Celia Hindmarch
August 2009

How to use this book

This book is a practical guide, illustrated with case studies taken from the experience of bereaved families and affected professionals, rather than an academic study. For most people it is more of a book to dip into than to read from cover to cover. Selected reading may be preferred according to interest and experience. All aspects of child death are covered.

Although case examples and statistics relate to the ages 0–19, it is recognised that the child status extends from prebirth to any age while parents are alive to grieve their loss.

There are three sections:
- ➤ the first deals with definitions and context, and relates theory to practice
- ➤ the second offers good practice guidelines related to various roles, client groups and situations
- ➤ and the third section gives an overview of different kinds of support.

The final chapter in this third section deals with the support which comes from inner resources.

The first three appendices offer information on resources for further support and reading. A fourth appendix has been added to develop guidelines on the use of geneograms in therapeutic work.

It is hoped that all readers will refer to the core messages contained in Chapter 4, *Guidelines for all*. These are simple though not always obvious. The most important ingredient in effective support is, of course, the relationship between the helper and bereaved. Whatever the nature of that relationship, whether health professional/patient, teacher/student, social worker/client, priest/parishioner, as friends or colleagues, common core conditions can be identified that help to create trust. While sensitivity cannot be taught, awareness of the issues can be developed and skills can be practised. The need for adequate support and supervision is strongly emphasised throughout as fundamental to professional good practice in this especially stressful area of bereavement care.

USE OF GENDER

For convenience, references are made to the dead child as male, and to the surviving sibling as female. At the risk of reinforcing stereotypes, adults are referred to in the predominant gender for the role or situation being considered.

USE OF STATISTICS

The tables and figures in Chapter 1 provide a simple picture of complex data, and are used to illustrate an overview of the incidence of child death.

Any variations in categories recorded compared with previous editions are due to different classifications of the cause of death.

Statistics from 2006 are the latest available figures across the board at the time of going to press.

SOURCES OF DATA

The data quoted in this book, mostly found in Chapter 2, are taken from the Office for National Statistics and relevant professional organisations.

About the author

Celia Hindmarch was the first manager and senior counsellor at the Alder Centre bereavement support project, Liverpool.

For a number of years she was a part-time tutor on counsellor training courses at Manchester University, and acted as consultant to Cheshire, Halton and Warrington local authorities regarding the support given to schools following critical incidents.

Acknowledgements

The author is indebted to all those who have contributed directly and indirectly to the book, and in particular to those who have shared their personal experience of grief on the death of a child.

Special thanks go to Alan Phillips, for sharing his vision of bereavement support and for introducing me to other contributors to this edition; to Mike O'Connor, who helped with the statistics; to Linda Machin, Sue Ashley and Nicholas Rheinberg, for helping to update other information; to Mike Johnson, for constructing the geneogram illustration; and to Gail Ashton, for generously sharing her research findings.

*This book is dedicated
to all our children*

SECTION 1

Theory and practice

CHAPTER 1

Incidence and characteristics of child death

'We find a place for what we lose. Although we know that after such a loss the acute stage of mourning will subside, we also know that we shall remain inconsolable and will never find a substitute. No matter what may fill the gap, even if it be filled completely, it nevertheless remains something else.'

Letters of Sigmund Freud (1961)

When my son Paul was killed in a road accident, a week after starting his first job, I didn't see that I had anything in common with younger parents who had lost a baby. But when I have heard such parents talking in a group I recognise the same pain. I feel so sorry for those parents. At least we had our son for 19 years.

Dave

Although this book covers many different situations involving the death of a child, all of them heartbreaking, it is important to remember that it is now a comparatively rare event in the Western world. Thankfully, most children recover from their accidents or illnesses nowadays. Modern health-care and technology ensure that most childhood diseases can be cured or controlled.

But some children do die. In 2006, the deaths of children aged 0–19 in England and Wales totalled 9505 (*see* Table 1.1) or 5903 excluding stillbirths (*see* Table 1.2). The impact of child death is out of all proportion to its incidence, in terms of the number of people affected and the severity of the effects.

TABLE 1.1 Number of child deaths (age 0–19 years) by cause in England and Wales, 2006

Category of death	Number	Percent
Sudden and accidental death		
sudden death, cause unknown (inc. SIDS)	187	2.0
road vehicle/transport accidents	512	5.4
other accidents	61	0.6
Totals	**760**	**8.0**
Natal deaths (excluding SIDS)		
stillbirth	3602	37.9
neonatal deaths <28 days	2345	24.7
Totals	**5947**	**62.6**
Death from illness/disease incl.		
mental and behaviour disorders	**1751**	**18.4**
Death from congenital conditions and those		
arising from pregnancy/birth incl.	556	5.8
abnormal clinical findings	246	2.6
Totals	**802**	**8.4**
Socially difficult deaths		
suicide/intentional harm	83	0.8
assault/murder	48	0.5
undetermined intent incl. drug misuse	124	1.3
Totals	**245**	**2.6**
Total of major categories	**9505**	**100.00**

Sources: Series DH2 Mortality Statistics: cause
Series DH3 Mortality Statistics: childhood, infant and perinatal
Health Statistics Quarterly 3
DR06 Mortality Statistics: deaths registered Office for National Statistics

Notes: SIDS = sudden infant death syndrome
2006 data is using ICD10; these are the codes and figures taken from DR06

TABLE 1.2 Total number of child deaths from all causes in England and Wales 2006

Sex	Under 1 year	1–4 years	5–9 years	10–14 years	15–19 years	0–19 years
Male	1863	292	187	261	844	3447
Female	1505	267	135	168	381	2456
Total	3368	559	322	429	1225	5903

Sources: Series DH2 Mortality Statistics: cause
DR06 Mortality Statistics: deaths registered
Office for National Statistics

THE DEATH OF A CHILD IS DIFFERENT FROM OTHER BEREAVEMENTS

Those who have lost a parent, a spouse and a child will invariably describe their grief for the child as the most painful, enduring and difficult to survive. For emergency services personnel, the death of a child is the casualty they most dread having to deal with. For medical and nursing staff, there is a special sense of failure and frustration when a child dies.

The enduring pain of losing a child cannot be measured, so that it is not possible to say that it is more or less painful to lose a child suddenly or after

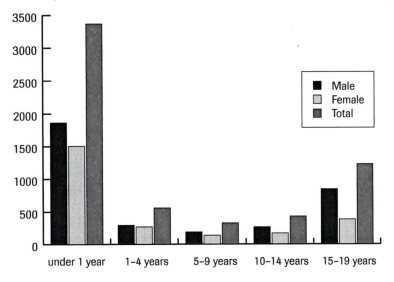

FIGURE 1.1 Child deaths (age 0–19) from any cause in England and Wales 2006 (excluding stillbirths)

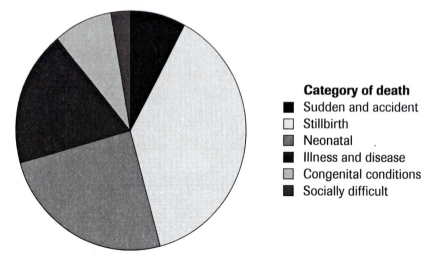

FIGURE 1.2 Categories of death in children (age 0–19) in England and Wales 2006

a long, debilitating illness; nor can it be assumed that the age of the child determines the intensity of the emotions (*see* Figure 1.1).

Clearly the mortality risk is highest in the first year of life, and boys outnumber girls at all ages. This gender difference is particularly marked during adolescence, which is associated with experimental and risk-taking behaviours.

In terms of adjustment, parents of older children have the benefit of more positive memories to draw on, although in another sense they have more to lose, having built up a relationship with the child in its own right.

However, it is certainly a different experience, with different factors to be taken into account. The characteristics of various situations will be considered by grouping the deaths into five main categories according to cause and circumstance (*see also* Table 1.1 and Figure 1.2):

➤ sudden and accidental deaths
➤ prenatal and perinatal loss
➤ death from illness
➤ death from congenital conditions
➤ socially difficult deaths.

Case studies are included to highlight certain characteristics, with the approval of the families concerned.

SUDDEN AND ACCIDENTAL DEATHS

Cot death

'Cot death' is the generic term used to describe the sudden, unexpected death of an apparently healthy baby. In about one-third of these cases, the post-mortem discovers an adequate cause to explain the death, such as an overwhelming infection. For the remaining two-thirds, no cause of death can be found and the death is certified as *sudden infant death syndrome* (SIDS). In either case, no-one could have foreseen or prevented the death.

Extensive research has pointed to a number of tenuous coincidental factors for SIDS in both baby and environment, but these are not identified causes. The lack of explanation feeds the mythology associated with this tragic death: Ancient Sumerians believed the baby was stolen by evil spirits; the Bible records a woman's child dying in the night 'because she overlaid it' (1 *Kings* 3:19); some East European countries still routinely record unexplained infant deaths as infanticide.

Facts and figures

Incidence

Variations that occur in the figures for cot death in any given year depend on which definitions are used, the age range, and on what appears on the death certificate. While the Office for National Statistics gives the figure of 187 as the number of sudden infant deaths in 2006 in England and Wales, the Foundation for the Study of Infant Deaths (FSID) estimates the figure to be 281. Whichever figure is taken, the important fact to note is that the number of deaths continues to fall after the dramatic drop in the rate that followed the Reduce the Risk campaign launched in 1991. Since then the FSID estimates a reduction of over 70%.

The Reduce the Risk campaign was based on the identification of certain factors that are *influential* rather than *causal*, and the FSID now promotes the following advice.

➤ Cut smoking in pregnancy – fathers too! And don't let anyone smoke in the same room as your baby.
➤ Place your baby on the back to sleep (and not on the front or side).
➤ Do not let your baby get too hot, and keep your baby's head uncovered.
➤ Place your baby with their feet to the foot of the cot, to prevent them wriggling down under the covers, or use a baby sleepbag.
➤ Never sleep with your baby on a sofa or armchair.

➤ The safest place for your baby to sleep is in a crib or cot in a room with you for the first six months.
➤ It is *especially* dangerous for your baby to sleep in your bed if you (or your partner):
  ➢ are a smoker, even if you never smoke in bed or at home
  ➢ have been drinking alcohol
  ➢ take medication or drugs that make you drowsy
  ➢ feel very tired
  or if your baby:
  ➢ was born before 37 weeks
  ➢ weighed less than 2.5 kilograms or 5.5 lb at birth.
➤ Settling your baby to sleep (day and night) with a dummy can reduce the risk of cot death, even if the dummy falls out while your baby is asleep.
➤ Breastfeed your baby. Establish breastfeeding before starting to use a dummy.

Age and circumstances

Cot death happens most frequently in the first six months of life, with a peak at two to three months. The rate drops sharply after six months, to become increasingly uncommon in the second year of life. Babies who die suddenly and unexpectedly are typically found dead in their cots in the morning, but some die in the pram, the car, or even in their parents' arms. There are no symptoms, although some babies – perhaps coincidentally – will have had the 'snuffles' in the preceding days.

Males are more at risk than females, as are twins, preterm and low-weight babies. Cot deaths occur in all social classes, although there is a higher incidence among babies born in disadvantaged families, to young mothers, to mothers who have a short interpregnancy interval, and those who do not present for antenatal care.

Legal procedures

A doctor has to confirm that the baby is dead, either at home or at hospital. As the death is sudden and unexpected, the doctor has by law to inform the coroner, or the procurator fiscal in Scotland, who will order a post-mortem examination.

A senior investigation officer will attend all sudden infant deaths, and is often from the Child Abuse Investigation Team. Since 2008 legislation has been in place that requires medical and forensic professionals to work together in investigating the death, including a joint home visit and a case conference to review all the evidence. The baby will have a post-mortem examination carried out by a paediatric pathologist on the instructions of the coroner.

For further information on what happens immediately after a sudden and unexpected death, *see* the booklet *When a Baby Dies Suddenly and Unexpectedly* produced by the Foundation for the Study of Infant Deaths, as part of their useful range of publications (*see* Appendix A for FSID contact details).

CASE STUDY

Tom was a bonny nine-pound baby at birth. At seven months he developed a chest infection, which the GP treated with antibiotics. A week later, when Tom seemed fully recovered, the family woke one morning to find him still and lifeless in his cot.

Tom's distraught parents, Dave and Sue, knew immediately he was dead, which was confirmed by their GP, who was first on the scene. After prescribing a sedative for Sue, he left with what seemed to the parents as undue haste. They later discovered that he had hurried home to check his seven-month-old baby girl before going to the surgery to look at Tom's notes to see whether he had missed something.

Meanwhile the police had arrived and completed their investigations with sensitivity. Most importantly for Sue, no-one tried to take Tom from her arms until she was ready to let him go. After a brief separation, while Sue and Dave followed Tom in the ambulance (although they wish now they had gone with him) they were reunited at the hospital.

'The staff were wonderful', Sue recalls. 'A nurse brought Tom in to us holding him close, as if he was still alive, treating him with respect. It meant a lot to us that someone said how beautiful he was, and a couple of the staff sat and cried with us. There was no rush.'

They had to leave Tom for the post-mortem examination over the weekend, but were welcomed whenever they returned to hold him again. Tom was home for two days before the funeral, an important time for the parents and for Tom's six-year-old brother Graeme, who read his book of nursery rhymes to the baby as his way of saying goodbye. Dave and Sue thought it best that three-year-old Michael did not see Tom, but with hindsight now wish they had allowed this, as Michael suffered awful fantasies of what Tom looked like. Fortunately there were photographs to allay his fears.

Sue was left with the overwhelming guilt of knowing that Tom died as she and Dave were sleeping in the same room. 'It took over three years to accept that I couldn't have done anything – and I still find it difficult.'

Death by accident

A major cause of accidental death in children is road traffic accidents (RTAs), where the child may be a pedestrian or passenger, and in later adolescence may be the driver of the vehicle. Other accident situations include death by drowning, choking, burning, falling and poisoning. The death may be immediate or as a result of injuries, and the child's body is likely to be damaged externally and sometimes severely maimed.

Whether or not other family members are involved in the accident, they will be suffering the effects of trauma. Extreme reactions of shock, disbelief and anger can be frightening and difficult for those in attendance.

Denial and evidence

Denial of what has happened is a natural defence and initially helps the traumatised system to cope. However, if the denial persists, the bereaved person will suffer from extreme anxiety and risks long-term mental health problems. Facing reality requires unambiguous explanation and evidence, and ultimately seeing is believing. The need to view the body or photographs of the deceased has been recorded by those who have worked with the relatives of disaster victims.

These were some of the conclusions reached by Janet Haddington after counselling families who lost a loved one in the sinking of the *Marchioness* in 1989 when, after the first two days, visual identifications of drowned relatives was first discouraged and then disallowed by the coroner's officers:

> 'The police should understand that identification may not be the sole reason for relatives wishing to view bodies. The bereaved also need to be clearly informed that photographs have been taken and will be made available at any stage in the future should seeing them feel helpful. The bereaved also need to be informed that once the body is released to the funeral director

they have the right to view. The manner in which some bereaved have been denied access to view the body has led to long-lasting anger and protracted grief.'

The use of the word 'denied' here is interesting, suggesting that professionals may seek to protect others from pain as a way of denying their own. Sometimes the mother is excluded from seeing the body in the belief that she is not strong enough to cope and may become hysterical.

Legal proceedings
The difficulty of dealing with intense grief reactions is exacerbated by legal proceedings, which may take months or even years to complete.

Accidental death requires a coroner's inquest to establish the cause of death. Where a person has been charged with murder, manslaughter, causing death by reckless driving or infanticide, the inquest is adjourned until the conclusion of the criminal proceedings. The evidence of witnesses and the results of police investigations will not be known until then, leaving parents in an anguish of uncertainty. It helps if the police keep them informed and if the coroner prepares them for the inquest, but too often they feel doubly victimised by an adversarial legal system that excludes them. In the case of a road traffic accident death that leads to a criminal charge and trial, parents desperately want the offender to admit responsibility and show regret. Sadly, the inevitable process of prosecution and defence makes this almost impossible. Most parents seek reparation, not retribution.

However, sentences for convictions of careless, reckless or dangerous driving leave the family and community feeling that a child's life is held cheap. The same applies to amounts paid as compensation.

Insensitive or intrusive media coverage will intensify the effects of the trauma.

CASE STUDY

Seventeen-year-old Kevin was a cheerful and popular lad with a sense of fun and adventure. While waiting for the train home one Saturday night, Kevin and his mates explored the goods area of the station and climbed on top of a wagon. Kevin touched the overhead electric wires and was killed outright.

Kevin's mother Betty was called home from her night-shift by the news that Kevin had been involved in an accident. Fearing the worst, she arrived home to find that her husband Kenny had already been taken away by the police. Her telephone enquiries to the local hospitals and police stations all drew a blank, and she was left in an agony of not knowing what had happened. Meanwhile, at the railway station, Kenny was told by the British Transport Police how Kevin had died, and was advised not to see his body. The officer who gave this advice had not seen Kevin himself, but assumed the body to be badly burned. Kenny identified Kevin from his watch and ring.

Back home, Betty's fears were confirmed when one of Kevin's friends who had witnessed the accident returned to his home a few doors away. She was angry and distressed to be separated from Kenny at the time they most needed to be together.

On his return, Kenny told Betty what he knew, and they comforted each other and their daughters as best they could.

They struggled with dreadful fantasies of what Kevin looked like and were anxious to know exactly what had happened. Two days after the accident they were shocked to read a tabloid newspaper report of the tragedy prefaced by the headline 'Fried Alive . . .' They were upset to read that British Rail were concerned about the boys trespassing.

Before the funeral, the undertaker heard the tentative note in the parents' question: 'Would you advise us to see him?' He replied that it was up to them, but they might prefer to remember Kevin as he was. They were frightened to do otherwise than heed his advice. Consequently they did not know what they were burying; later, Kenny owned his vision of 'a burnt head of a matchstick'. Betty simply could not believe Kevin was dead. It had all been a ghastly mistake and one day he would just turn up at the back door, having been away on one of his army courses.

At the same time, Betty was inconsolable. She began to resent Kevin's friends and was convinced they were hiding the true story from her. She was advised not to go to the inquest, some four months later, as being 'too upsetting' for her. Kenny attended, and watched helplessly as photographs of Kevin's dead body were passed among the jury – photographs that he did not know existed.

Over three years later, Betty was still angry and bitter. 'I'm left with this void. If I had seen him, I would have known he was dead, instead of waiting for him to come home, which is what I still do.'

Disaster

The deaths of children caught up in a disaster, as at Aberfan, Hillsborough and Lockerbie, awaken themes of violence and senselessness. Where there are many deaths together, the intensity of the shared grief is overwhelming, and extremely difficult to resolve. This is compounded by the protracted legal battles to determine responsibility, and it is bitterly resented when no-one is held accountable. Fears of litigation, compensation awards and individual job dismissal make it almost impossible for anyone to show the regret and remorse the parents badly want to hear expressed.

There is usually an overwhelming need to be with others who have experienced or been affected by the disaster. New identities are forged: as casualties, as survivors, as bereaved, as helpers. Multiple losses affect the whole community for many years after the event that has somehow defined its members differently. Gaynor, who survived the Aberfan coal tip disaster in 1966 which killed her brother and sister, remembers some of the after-effects as follows:

> 'After the disaster the surviving children weren't allowed to play in the street in case it upset other parents. We all felt guilty we were alive. We didn't feel like survivors. I have always felt insecure and this is the reason I have changed jobs and house so often. It has destroyed a lot of people's lives. Most of the survivors I know are divorced and have lived very unsettled lives.'
>
> (*The Guardian*, 23 March 1999)

Bombings which have killed innocent children in Northern Ireland, notably at Omagh in 1998, in blatant disregard of the ceasefire, have left lasting scars emotionally as well as physically. Even those bombings that claim no children, as in the Docklands, or that involve no deaths at all, as in Manchester, may affect the security of children who see their homes or schools damaged.

Miraculously only one child and three adults perished as a result of the *Jupiter* sea disaster in 1988, when nearly 400 children embarked on an educational cruise from the port of Piraeus in Greece. Ten years later the trip coordinator has compiled the memories of some of the children and parents. The experience of the ship sinking and the struggle to survive marked the end of a carefree existence for those involved. One parent said: 'I sent away a child and got back a stranger'. An Institute of Psychiatry interim report (1996) found that 52% of 168 *Jupiter* survivors interviewed had experienced symptoms of post-traumatic stress disorder (PTSD); that 14% continued to experience PTSD symptoms for more than five years; that 9% of the group have attempted suicide since the disaster; and that there are significant differences in academic performance compared to contemporaries.

It is important to note also the amazingly strong bonds which can hold people together after disasters, and the inner resources which children can call upon. The *Jupiter* accounts are full of examples of calm self-discipline. When another boat carrying a party of young people hit disaster a year later – the *Marchioness* on the River Thames in London – young friends on the accompanying sister ship *Hurlingham* displayed extraordinary courage in their attempts to save lives.

PRENATAL AND PERINATAL LOSS
Miscarriage

Miscarriage is also known as spontaneous abortion. Nobody knows the true incidence, as many early miscarriages are not reported, but it is estimated that over 20% of all clinically confirmed pregnancies end in miscarriage before 20 weeks' gestation. Allowing for the reality that some women feel relieved to miscarry in the event of an unwanted pregnancy, miscarriage still accounts for the highest incidence of child loss. After the age of viability, set at 24 weeks' gestation in the UK, the fetus is regarded as a baby and its death described as a stillbirth. But for most parents, and particularly for the mother, the growing mass of cells has always been a baby. With the aid of ultrasound scans, parents can now see the growing shape and movements of their baby long before the mother can feel it move inside her.

Early miscarriage means there is nothing to say goodbye to, and no ritual to help make the loss a reality. Anguish and guilt may derive from not knowing what happened to the fetus, which becomes hospital property. Fortunately, growing awareness has enabled health professionals to acknowledge these anxieties. Mothers are now encouraged to see and hold a formed baby, however small, and many chaplains will arrange some kind of funeral long before the law requires it. Most parents will appreciate a scan picture, if one is available, as evidence that their baby existed.

Late miscarriage means the baby has died nearer to a viable age (redefined by the Stillbirth (Definition) Act 1992 as 24 weeks' gestation) and is legally entitled to a funeral. Medical terms such as 'placental insufficiency' and 'cervical incompetence' encourage the mother's feeling that she is to blame. The later the loss, the greater the attachment will have been between mother and baby, and to a lesser extent between father and baby, so that grief reactions are likely to be more intense. The importance of naming the baby, spending time to say goodbye, and a proper and dignified ritual, have all been established as helpful for healthy grieving. Photographs are usually treasured by the parents, and are helpful to other family members such as grandparents and siblings who were not able to see the baby.

CASE STUDY

Faye and Denis always planned to have two children. They hoped for a girl and a boy. Eighteen months after having Michael, Faye lost her second baby, Deborah, at 20 weeks' gestation:

> 'I was sure she had been dead for a couple of weeks, but at first no-one seemed to take me seriously when I said I knew something was wrong. I didn't even see her, and felt guilty afterwards. I didn't like to ask what happened to her little body, but I guessed. When I went back on the ward nobody knew what to say to me and I couldn't wait to get home.'

Having been told that she might not be able to carry another baby to term, Faye was apprehensive when she became pregnant again eight years later. She lost Jane at 17 weeks, but this was a very different experience.

> 'Denis came with me for the scan, which confirmed the worst, and he stayed with me when they induced labour. Jane was so tiny she could fit in your hand. We held her and had some photographs taken and the sister asked if we wanted the chaplain to come. We knew she couldn't baptise her but she did a sort of blessing, which meant a lot to us. Jane even had a proper little funeral service, and we can visit the Petal Garden at the local crematorium where the ashes of all premature babies are scattered. I just wish we could have done the same for Deborah.'

Termination

In 2006 the total number of recorded pregnancy terminations in England and Wales was 193 737. A small number of these terminations were medically advised, because of fetal abnormality or because of risk to the pregnant woman's life. The vast majority were requested on the grounds that continuance of the pregnancy would jeopardise the physical or mental health of the pregnant woman or her existing children (Abortion Statistics 2006, Office for National Statistics).

Requested termination

Termination as a solution to unwanted pregnancy may be sought for a variety of reasons. In the younger age group, a girl's pregnancy may be at odds with her maturational and educational needs, it may be the result of forced sex or it may be the consequence of trying to get psychological needs met. For an older woman, there may be a conflict with other priorities at that time. She may fear that this baby will impose emotional, mental or physical demands that will be damaging to herself or her family. At any age, she may want the baby but is under pressure from family or partner not to continue with the pregnancy, and may lack the support she needs. Whatever the circumstances, termination is likely to be a negative choice with some level of regret. It may be necessary to deny this conflict of feelings in order to go through with the decision. The medical assessment that follows a request for termination subjects the woman to the kind of scrutiny that is not required of a woman who decides to have a child. Pre-abortion counselling is unlikely to uncover ambivalence or regret in women who do not feel able to make free choices.

Medically advised termination

If there is evidence that a baby will be born with a significant abnormality, either because of a congenital condition or because the baby has been exposed to potential damage, or if the continued pregnancy puts the mother's health at serious risk, then a termination will be offered to the mother. If she decides to terminate on the basis of uncertain risks, she may never know whether the baby would have been all right, and the responsibility of making such a painful decision will weigh heavily. Even when the choice is obvious, the mother is likely to feel guilt and a sense of failure. Again, these feelings may need to be denied at the time in favour of logic and common sense.

The termination of an abnormal fetus is experienced as a double bereavement, compounded by feelings of guilt and inadequacy that the baby was 'faulty'. Whatever the reason for the termination, the feelings of loss may be intense. The grief for what might have been is often underestimated, particularly when the termination has been voluntary and a matter of painful choice.

Stillbirth

In 2006, 3602 stillbirths were registered in England and Wales (*see* Figure 1.1). This figure has risen since 1992, when the Stillbirth (Definition) Act lowered the definition age for stillbirth from 28 to 24 weeks gestation. There can be few more distressing experiences than to give birth to a dead baby, or be witness to this cruel loss. The stillness of a new-born baby is a tragic juxtaposition of life and death.

Although a baby who has not been born alive has no status in law, a case might go to the coroner if the act of a third person brought about the death of the baby (or the mother and therefore the baby) as in an attack or car crash.

The process of registering the stillbirth is very painful for most parents, though for some it can provide an opportunity for confronting the reality of what has happened. Parents are issued with a certificate of registration.

SANDS (the Stillbirth and Neonatal Death Society) has done much to raise awareness about the need of parents to say goodbye to their baby, and many hospitals now have a room or suite available within the maternity unit but away from the ward.

Neonatal death

Neonatal means newly born, and defines the period from birth to 28 days. This overlaps with the term 'perinatal', which applies to the period between the viability time of gestation (24 weeks) and the first seven days after birth, so for that first week the two words can be used synonymously. There were 2345 neonatal deaths in England and Wales in 2006 (*see* Table 1.1). Some causes of neonatal death are common to stillbirth: abnormal development, premature delivery and complications during labour. The baby may have been born without the necessary capacity for survival, which is usually anticipated before the birth, or unexpected problems during labour may harm an otherwise healthy baby. In the latter case the mother may be heavily sedated, have undergone an emergency caesarean section, and be quite unwell after the birth. Her own incapacity can have important consequences if the baby dies before she can relate to him.

The baby's initial attachments, however, are to machines and tubes, and the parents' first sight of their baby surrounded by technology and protected by a wall of plastic can be frightening. There is usually an intense longing to hold the baby, which may be frustrated until the baby dies. Neonatal Unit staff encourage parents to handle the baby whenever possible, and share the baby's care. However, some parents withdraw emotionally and physically from the baby in anticipation of their loss.

This can be a source of acute feelings of guilt later on, and is distressing to the staff and other parents on the unit. The loss of a twin, when emotional energies are split between the surviving twin and the dying twin, is especially poignant.

The parents have experienced their baby as having an independent life. That life is valued, however short, and parents will specify hours and minutes when describing their loss. There is often a tragic sense of helplessness, for both parents and staff, as the fight for life is lost. The primary nurse, the consultant and the spiritual care advisor may assume great significance for the parents, as being the main characters in the baby's short life.

DEATH FROM ILLNESS
Malignant disease

The diagnosis of childhood cancer is not the death sentence it is often presumed to be, and the majority of children with the most common form of leukaemia have a good prognosis of long-term survival. Treatments and therapies for cancers and blood disorders are often painful and distressing, involving disfiguring side-effects such as hair loss from chemotherapy and puffy weight gain from steroids. Periods of remission give rise to hope and optimism, but as successive treatments fail for those with a poor prognosis, there is time to prepare for the inevitable outcome.

Some parents and families do plan accordingly, and provide many varied life-experiences for their child's remaining months or years, such as trips abroad and visits to Disneyland. Others do not or cannot even talk about the future and cope by maintaining denial to the end. In either case the question remains whether it is ever possible to feel prepared for the reality of the death when it occurs.

Stories are legion of the courage of these children in approaching death. The home services provided by specialist Macmillan nurses and Sargent cancer care workers can help to normalise the family's life and facilitate the child's death at home wherever possible.

CASE STUDY

David was 15 months old when his parents were told the diagnosis to explain a persistent lump (and his mother's intuition) that he was seriously unwell: a stage four neuroblastoma, with a very poor prognosis for recovery. Sue and John remember the compassion of the consultant at their local hospital who was clearly upset to tell them this bad news. David was transferred to the nearest paediatric hospital, Alder Hey in Liverpool, for the specialist treatment he needed. This was one of the worst times: arriving at a strange place at the weekend, when the ward was eerily quiet, and suddenly feeling totally out of control, shocked and angry that this was happening to their child.

Sue's philosophy is to face things head-on, and John's recent experience of losing both parents in an atmosphere of secrecy and denial made them both determined to be open about David's illness. They appreciated the Alder Hey consultant answering their questions honestly, balancing hope with realism. They came to feel part of a team, working together with medical and nursing staff, social worker and play therapist, and became part of a ward culture that enabled parents to support each other.

There followed a regime of chemotherapy, to which David responded well, with a week in hospital and two weeks at home. Sue and John readily responded to the Sargent social worker's advice to include Jane, their three-year-old daughter, in what was going on. As a result, all three of them would sometimes stay with David on the ward at weekends. Otherwise Sue and John took it in turns to be with him while the other maintained a secure base for Jane. Throughout his illness, David's quality of life was high, and they were able to function as a normal family for much of the time. After six months, the time was judged right for surgery to remove the primary tumour. The immediate improvement in David's condition after the operation gave new hope – only to be dashed within weeks when tests confirmed that the cancerous growth had returned. This was the darkest hour for Sue and John, with the realisation that time was running out. After David reacted badly to one last-chance experimental treatment, they felt he had had enough, and active treatment was stopped.

David died at home, without pain, two weeks before his second birthday, hours after watching his favourite Postman Pat videos together with his family. Sue describes it as an extraordinarily peaceful day.

Acute illness

Viral infections such as meningitis can overwhelm a child very quickly. By the time the parents become alarmed by symptoms and call the doctor or take the child to hospital, the child's condition is likely to have worsened rapidly. When the child dies, perhaps within a day or two, the loss is experienced as a sudden death, and the parents are caught in a nightmare of disbelief. Typically parents will blame themselves for not alerting the doctor earlier and so, maybe, reducing the chances of recovery. The mysterious power of an invisible killer disease that can strike without warning lends itself to quite irrational conclusions: parents may become convinced that a playmate was carrying the infection, or that a recent visit to the shops was somehow connected. Fears for the safety of surviving children are likely to run high and lead to overprotective attitudes. The family too may suffer from others' irrational beliefs that it is somehow contaminated by such tragic fortune and thus better avoided.

DEATH FROM CONGENITAL CONDITIONS
Cystic fibrosis

This is the most common genetically inherited life-threatening disorder.

However, life-expectancy has increased steadily as symptom treatment has improved; many children with cystic fibrosis now survive into adulthood. Careful exercise and management can sustain a near-normal lifestyle for much of the time.

As the children and parents are in and out of hospital over a number of years, strong attachments form with hospital staff. Hospital and community nurses become part of an extended family, and they come to see the family as friends more than patients. Children who want to talk about their condition may protect their parents from distress by talking to a trusted nurse – perhaps at night when the child is alone and has time to think. The staff are therefore closely involved in the child's life and death.

Heart deformities

Over one-third of hospital child deaths relate to congenital heart conditions, although in a few cases the heart deformity develops as the result of a viral infection. Six children per 1000 are born with some kind of heart abnormality: of these, one-third die soon after birth, and one-third will require surgery. Although the child has had a chronically sick condition, the death is usually experienced as sudden, as most typically occur in surgery and at a young age.

Although the parents are told the risks of survival, the faith required to hand over their child to the surgeon suspends any realistic view. The shock, disbelief and anger that parents experience are compounded by the fatal operation taking place when the child was in the best of health (to optimise the chances of coming through). Thus the parents may have brought in a comparatively healthy child who was skipping down the ward one day, and is dead the next.

One important consequence of this pattern of events is the guilt that parents feel that they were not with their child when he died, and the heavy sense of responsibility that, in consenting to this operation, they virtually signed a death warrant. Anger towards the surgeon and the hospital is often extreme, and more parents are resorting to litigation. This natural anger is overwhelming for parents if there is any doubt about the surgeon's competence or assessment of risk, as featured in the Bristol Royal Infirmary inquiry held between 1998 and 1999.

CASE STUDY

Newborn baby Clare's feeding difficulties and a blueness around the lips alerted maternity staff that something was badly wrong. John and Maureen, her parents, were told there was a slim chance of her surviving the necessary surgery to insert a shunt. But she did survive, and came through major surgery at 18 months with flying colours. John remembers that they were totally oblivious to the risks at that time – perhaps because they didn't want to know – and had absolute faith in the surgeon.

To all outward appearances Clare grew up a very normal little girl: she went to a normal school, joined the Brownies, Guides and majorettes, and John taught her to swim. But she couldn't run about like other children, and her parents always had to be extra vigilant to make sure she didn't overdo things. And as she got older, the need for more corrective surgery grew with her.

'It was rather like living with a gas leak', John recalls. 'You don't realise the danger until someone comes in from outside and brings it to your notice. We didn't see how much Clare had deteriorated.'

It wasn't until the last year of Clare's life that John and Maureen realised that she might die. Meeting other parents through the Association for Children with Heart Disorders opened their eyes. With no other options left, Clare faced major surgery again at the age of ten-and-a-half years, and this time she did not come through.

'Something inside me just knew she wouldn't make it', says John. 'We really started grieving for her from the time we were told of the operation – like picking up a newspaper dated three months later. But it was still an enormous shock to lose her.'

Neurodegenerative disorders

There are literally hundreds of genetically inherited life-threatening diseases, some very rare, which are mostly metabolic in origin. The most common of these conditions include the dystrophies and Batten's disease. The principle feature of these neurodegenerative disorders is the progressive deterioration of the neurological system over weeks, months or years. This often includes a distressing deterioration of mental faculty.

The timing of the diagnosis varies, but typically an apparently well child will develop non-specific symptoms such as epileptic fits, a squint or an awkward gait. At first the degeneration may be slow, and parents can suffer years of struggle and worry, perhaps being labelled as overanxious by the medical profession. As the symptoms increase and the condition worsens, tests lead to a diagnosis. The label makes no difference to the outcome, and the parents will be told that the condition is life-threatening. The bereavement starts here, and some anticipatory grieving will begin as the child's functioning becomes progressively worse.

Parents are desperate to know the prognosis, and most will ask: 'How long has he got?' Time limits and future plans become all-consuming preoccupations. No-one can give a confident prediction of life expectancy, as the progression of the disease can remain on a plateau for several years. Care of the increasingly disabled child becomes the focus of family life, and respite care provides both a lifeline and a potential source of guilt for parents who become physically and emotionally exhausted.

Many of these children die in their early teenage years, usually from an infection which the debilitated system is unable to resist.

After such a death families are vulnerable to wounding remarks such as 'all for the best' and 'blessing in disguise'. Parents lose a lifestyle of care and a social network as well as their beloved child.

SOCIALLY DIFFICULT DEATHS

Some deaths carry an element of social stigma, presenting an added difficulty for families coming to terms with their grief. Murder, suicide, deaths associated with anorexia, substance misuse, AIDS, neglect and abuse evoke highly emotive responses at a social level. Such deaths are difficult to talk about, subject to myth and misunderstanding, and reduce the level of sympathetic support forthcoming in other situations. Bereaved families are thus likely to be further isolated.

Murder

The wounds may never heal for parents of murder victims. There may be an agonising period of uncertainty between the discovery that the child is missing and finding the body, then again before the perpetrator is apprehended. If the body is not found, or is mutilated beyond recognition, the reality of the death is hard to reconcile. The legal process then takes over in a way that leaves the family feeling doubly victimised. Sensitive police handling of the case will take into account the importance of the family being kept as fully informed as possible. The parents are tormented by imaginings of their child's final violation, and their private grief is likely to be invaded by the media.

Suicide

Suicide is perhaps the biggest taboo of all, particularly in adolescence. It is hard to accept that a youngster, with all of life's potential before him, should choose to end it. Suicide is a massive rejection of the parents who conceived and nurtured that life. The act of self-destruction, whether or not it was intended to result in death, may well happen at a time when family relationships are fraught and ambivalent.

Denial is an understandable defence against the burden of guilt and sense of failure that threaten to overwhelm the parents. Coroners often collude with this and return an open verdict if at all possible in order to spare the family's feelings. In fact, the uncertainty that follows an open verdict may hinder the grieving. As long as the parents can harbour the belief that there may have been a third party involved, or that an experiment went dreadfully wrong, they will engage all their energies in exploiting every theory that avoids facing reality.

In any case, the experience of social isolation is likely to be the same, adding a sense of shame to the guilt and responsibility. The stresses on parents and siblings are enormous, and suicidal thoughts of joining the dead youngster are commonly experienced. The expression of such dark feelings brings some relief, and contact with other families who have been through this ordeal can be reassuring.

Schools and colleges find it very difficult to deal with the suicide of a student. The events are usually shrouded in mystery and rumour, and a fear of copycat actions often prevents the staff from acknowledging the death openly. The myth that talking about suicide encourages others to feel suicidal still persists, while the healthiest outcome is for youngsters to express their feelings of shock and fear. (*See* Chapter 6, pp 133–6, and Chapter 8, pp 177–9.)

CASE STUDY

During the last three months of his life, Simon had lost his job and written off his first car. In spite of these setbacks he did not appear to be depressed, and his family had no hint beforehand of his suicidal feelings. On a bitterly cold winter day he waited until his mother went out with the dogs, left a note for his parents, took some rope from the loft and made his way to a park behind a nearby pub. There he hanged himself from a tree in an area where he used to play as a child.

By the time the note was found and the police called, Simon's body had been discovered and taken to hospital. At first the police said there was still hope of the paramedics reviving him when they knew he was dead, which later caused much resentment from the family. There was an agonising two-hour wait before Simon's parents and two older sisters were allowed to go to the hospital. The police were perceived as kind but when they attempted to talk to Simon's father on his own, Simon's mother felt hurt and demanded not to be left out. The family needed to be together and travelled to the hospital in the same car.

At the hospital the doctor who confirmed the death was experienced but cold and detached, and the family wished he had shown some feeling. The family found the nurses to be kind and considerate, and they were given as much time as they wanted with the body. Simon's older sister remembers being upset that his feet were not covered by the sheet.

Waiting for the inquest was a harrowing time, even though the suicide note left no doubt of the verdict. It read: 'Mum and Dad, I did something stupid today. So it is obvious my brain is not right or that I am not right. So I have gone to cure it for good. I love you very much, Simon.' Without any other explanation, the perplexed parents were deeply hurt by unfounded rumours that Simon had been thrown out of home, that he was on drugs, that he had 'got a girl into trouble'. They felt isolated by the implications that his home and family had been inadequate.

Substance misuse

Experimental use of drugs and other substances is widespread among young people, and in the UK almost universal as far as alcohol is concerned. The highest risk of accidental death occurs early on in the usage, when youngsters have low tolerance levels and are ignorant about the potentially lethal effects. It is believed that as many as a third of deaths from drug misuse occur as a result of the user's first experience. Ambivalent and somewhat hypocritical social attitudes towards drug-taking do not help. Drugs education programmes that aim to minimise risk by giving children the information they need to stay safe are not promoted, on the grounds that such information encourages substance misuse. Parents may find it very difficult to come to terms with their child's behaviour, which was concealed from them, and seek scapegoats to blame. Often the family gets labelled as somehow inadequate.

AIDS

HIV (Human Immunodeficiency Virus) which leads to AIDS (Acquired Immune Deficiency Syndrome) is transmitted through bodily fluids, principally blood, semen and vaginal fluids. In the case of children being infected with HIV the routes of transmission particular to them are believed to be while in the womb, during birth and breast feeding. Such is the stigma still attached to AIDS that most parents of these children are unable to share with others the true nature of their child's condition or cause of death.

Care issues

Deaths that are linked in some way to neglect of the child or to non-accidental injuries evoke strong emotions. They usually take place against a background of deprivation and inadequacy, and the majority are character-ised by some degree of domestic violence. If the child dies with some real degree of parental responsibility, the parents' grief is likely to be ignored by a society that condemns them. The support of other bereaved parents is not available to them, and expert psychiatric care may be indicated.

The professionals involved when a child dies through neglect or non-accidental injury may also be deeply affected. If the child has been on the 'at risk' register, the social worker and/or health visitor may have tried to develop trusting relationships with the parent(s) while carrying a heavy load of responsibility for the child's safety – an almost impossible psychological juggling act. This tension was well described by the head of Haringey Children's Services, Sharon Shoesmith, who was sacked along with five other staff as part of the fallout from the 'Baby P' case in 2008. The 17-month-old baby died as a result of terrible injuries at the hands of his mother, her boyfriend and a male lodger, after previous opportunities to take this child into care had been missed. The existence of the two men was apparently concealed from the social worker monitoring the baby's welfare, who was seeking to support a struggling mother seemingly welcoming her help. In the aftermath of the inquiries that followed the baby's death, the frontline staff and managers lost their jobs and reputations. They were inevitably vilified by the popular press.

The death of a baby born to a girl who is herself in care will have implications for her carers too.

Fostering

Children who have died while in the care of social services will have developed relationships with various professionals, notably their foster carers (*see* Dave and Carol's story, Chapter 10). Foster carers may be involved when a terminally ill child cannot be cared for within the birth family, for whatever reason, and will be faced with similar grief issues to the birth parents. Sometimes foster carers may be excluded from funeral arrangements made by the birth family, and their grief issues may go unrecognised.

ORGAN RETENTION

Revelations in the late 1990s that body parts of children had been retained for research purposes without the parents' knowledge or permission scandalised the nation. This practice was carried on in some hospitals over a number of years by a small number of rogue professionals, but did untold damage to the reputation of paediatric pathology in general.

Alder Hey Children's Hospital serving Merseyside and the north-west of England became the focus of these revelations in 1999, as a result of the practice of Professor Dick Van Velsen, a paediatric pathologist who had accumulated a vast collection of child body parts following post-mortem examinations. 'Body parts' is a term which includes slides and blocks of tissue samples as well as whole organs such as heart, brain and liver. There followed a 'reconciliation' process, which involved identifying organs and their release for interment. The remaining unidentified organs and tissues were interred at open funerals over a period of years.

Sir Michael Redfern was commissioned to investigate the organ retention scandal. *The Royal Liverpool Children's Enquiry: main report and evidence* (Redfern, 2001), which became known as the Redfern Report, was published in January 2001. This report was particularly critical of the practices of Van Velsen and recommended that the Crown Prosecution Service (CPS) be informed. However, the CPS concluded in 2004 that while there were grounds for criminal prosecution of Van Velsen, it was not advisable to proceed because it would be impossible to prove that retained organs were correctly labelled and identified. This was a crushing blow to parents who sought accountability and retribution. In June 2005 there was some small consolation in the guilty verdict found against Van Velsen by the General Medical Council, which meant that he would not be allowed to practise in the UK again.

On the one hand, it may be difficult for some people to appreciate the emotional impact on families faced with the knowledge that the body of the child they had buried or cremated was incomplete, and that some part of their child had been retained without their permission. This amounted to a huge betrayal of trust and generated justifiable anger. For those who had adjusted to their original loss, organ retention reawakened that loss and grief. Those who had never come to terms with their child's death were faced with their unresolved grief and complex psychological problems. On the other hand, the horrific images associated with organ retention led some people to overestimate the amount of psychological or even psychiatric help that would be needed. The manager of the Alder Centre at the time, Alan Phillips, argued against pathologising affected parents according to a medical model of disease, diagnosis and treatment. He pointed out that not everyone wanted or needed professional interventions:

> 'Let us not forget that one of the major criticisms of the Redfern Report arose from the overly paternalistic impositions of professionals working without the inclusion and consent of parents.'
>
> (from 'Light out of darkness' article published in *Healthcare Counselling and Psychotherapy Journal*, July 2006)

Alder Hey was not the only hospital where organ retention had taken place, but it attracted the most publicity. It was ironic that the same institution that had pioneered progressive services and preached parent inclusion was also vulnerable to the arrogant and unprofessional practice of organ retention.

Fortunately the hospital Trust could look to the Alder Centre, which exemplified parental participation and inclusion, to coordinate therapeutic support for affected families and hospital staff. The Centre introduced the Family Support Project, which offered an extension of existing services, including befriending, counselling, group support and the Child Death Helpline. Centre counsellors, in a setting one step removed from the hospital itself, acted as an emotional firewall for those who needed to express their outrage.

References

Foundation for the Study of Infant Deaths. *When a Baby Dies Suddenly and Unexpectedly.* London: FSID; 1988. Available at: www.thebabywebsite.com/article.72.When_a_baby_dies_suddenly_and_unexpectedly.htm (accessed 24 June 2009).

Redfern M. *The Royal Liverpool Children's Inquiry; main report and evidence.* London: The Stationery Office; 2001.

Phillips A. Light out of darkness: Alder Hey assessed. *Healthc Counsell Psychother J.* 2006; July; pp. 22–25.

Further reading

Phillips A. Handling emotions at work: Alder Hey assessed. *Healthc Counsell Psychother J.* 2007; January; pp. 21–24

CHAPTER 2

Features of grief and mourning when a child dies

'Grief fills the room up of my absent child
Lies in his bed, walks up and down with me
Puts on his pretty looks, repeats his words
Remembers me of all his gracious parts
Stuffs out his vacant garments with his form.'

Constance, on the death of her son Arthur
(*King John* Act III, Scene IV)

INTRODUCTION: STARTING FROM EXPERIENCE

'When my grandson died, some people thought I shouldn't be grieving the way I was. One person said that losing a child was no different to losing a much-loved partner or parent. I told her that if she ever lost a child or grandchild, to come back and tell me what she thinks then.' Diane

'Don't talk to me about the grieving process . . . What a ludicrously inappropriate phrase to define the mental, physical and emotional turmoil you are left to sort out after your child has died.' Marilyn

Both the grandmother and mother quoted here are expressing their frustration with the way society underestimates their experience of loss. They are saying that the death of a child *is* different from other bereavements, that this difference sets them apart from other people and that bereavement jargon is inadequate to describe the uniqueness of their experience and nature of their grief.

For professionals, too, there are special implications of dealing with the death of a child:

> 'I have had 20 years' experience as an accident and emergency nurse, and I can remember every child we've worked on and lost. I'm never prepared for that. I'm always drained afterwards, emotionally and psychologically. I just want to go home.' Jan

> 'I've been with the ambulance service over 13 years. Dealing with a child is totally different to an adult, and for me, cot death is more traumatic than anything else. I feel sick and totally useless.' Ron

Whether personally or professionally involved, the death of a child is seen as the most difficult loss to cope with. It is also seen as the most difficult death to talk about and anticipate. It is important to understand why this is so.

Theoretical concepts are formed in order to make sense of experience. Making sense of experience – of what is thought and felt internally as well as what happens externally – may be very helpful to the bereaved themselves. Equally, the search for understanding is driven by professionals asking questions such as: how can bereaved parents and families best be helped by others? When and what kind of intervention is indicated? Who might be most vulnerable?

Models of grief are not dreamed up out of the air. They rely on observation and empirical research, using individual experiences in comparative studies, to create some norms from the similarities and differences which emerge. Thus experience forms theory, and theory informs experience.

However, it is fair to say that conventional theories of grief have been found inadequate when it comes to the death of a child. This is partly due to the fact that the majority of bereavement research studies have concentrated on conjugal grief after the death of a spouse or partner. Perhaps more significantly, these models have rested on some basic assumptions which are now seen to be flawed, or certainly limited by their time and culture. Research developments at the end of the twentieth century and beginning of the twenty-first century challenge these assumptions, and they pay more attention to parental grief, child grief and social perspectives. Alternative and modified models are now available which bring together experience and theory with an exciting freshness, and these will be considered in this chapter. Specifically the concept of the *resolution of grief* will be challenged. First, the features of grief and mourning that inform our understanding of bereavement will be summarised.

THE DEVELOPMENT OF BEREAVEMENT THEORY

Bereavement has come to mean the loss by death of someone significant, although it originally referred to the marauding practices of bands of reavers many centuries ago, raiding the livestock of neighbouring clans. Thus, to be be-reaved implies being robbed or deprived of something or someone of value, so that one is necessarily poorer for the loss. To be deprived of someone of value implies attachment, and the degree of attachment will determine the degree of loss experienced, which leads to grief:

➤ *bereavement* is what happens
➤ *grief* is what one feels in reaction to the bereavement
➤ *mourning* is what one does to express grief.

The twentieth century, Western understanding of grief maintains that successful mourning means that the bereaved must disengage from the deceased. Continued attachment to the dead person is seen as denying the reality of the loss. This notion is traced to Freud (1917), with quotations such as the following to support it: 'When the work of mourning is completed the ego becomes free and uninhibited again'; and 'Mourning has quite a precise psychical task to perform: its function is to detach the survivor's hopes and memories from the dead.'

The British psychiatrist John Bowlby said that the important focus for understanding grief is what happens when attachments are threatened or broken, that is, strong emotional reactions occur automatically (Bowlby, 1969–80). When faced with loss, attachment behaviour is activated as a chain reaction of distress, anger and withdrawal, all geared towards retrieving the loss. This forms the pattern of the grieving process.

Bowlby's ideas about grief were consolidated and developed by another British psychiatrist, Colin Murray Parkes, via extensive studies of widows in the 1970s. Grief became increasingly understood as a predictable set of behaviours in response to the environment, and resolution of the grief was seen as getting through these reactions to the point where the attachment was dissolved and the reality of the loss finally accepted. These grief reactions have been variously described as parts or stages of a process, though Parkes himself prefers the concept of *phases*, and describes four phases of mourning (Parkes, 1972; Parkes and Brown, 1972).

The American psychologist William Worden, whose book *Grief Counselling and Grief Therapy*, (3rd edition 2003) is widely regarded as a standard text, adds to this model the concept of *tasks* of mourning which relate to each of the phases. These four phases, with their associated features and tasks, are summarised in Table 2.1.

TABLE 2.1 The four phases of grief

Phase	Features	Task
1 Denial	Shock, disbelief, sense of unreality	To accept the reality of the loss
2 Pain/distress	Hurt, anger, guilt, worthlessness, searching	To experience the pain of grief
3 Realisation	Depression, apathy, fantasy	To adjust to life without the deceased
4 Adjustment	Readiness to engage in new activities and relationships	To relocate emotional energy elsewhere

Worden (4e 2008)

Worden's emphasis on the tasks of mourning encourages both mourner and helper to recognise the potential for aiding the grief work in hand. At the same time the idea of task suggests a necessary degree of resolution before the next phase can be negotiated and the whole process can be successfully completed. However, Worden takes care to point out that many variable factors will influence an individual's progress through these phases, and that their culmination will not restore the mourner to a pre-grief state. It is also important to note that in later editions of his book, Worden revises Task 4 from *'withdraw emotional energy from the deceased and reinvest it in another relationship'* to *'emotionally relocate the deceased and move on with life'*. In particular, he takes into account here the difficulty bereaved parents have with the notion of emotional withdrawal from their children. In asking *When is mourning finished?* Worden seeks to acknowledge the ambiguity of the question while maintaining that there is such a thing as 'a completed grief reaction'.

When tasks of mourning are not completed, we are led inevitably to the notion of 'abnormal' grief reactions. Such a label relates to the medical model of grief that measures reactions as 'healthy' or 'pathological'. Nonconformity with behavioural norms is seen as denial of reality.

So, taking care to avoid such unhelpful language, I will attempt to summarise the conventional view of predictable grief reactions, what happens when they differ from the norm, and how they apply to the death of a child.

Predictable grief reactions

These are defined by Worden as both clinically predictable and common across the whole spectrum of the grieving experience. A broad range of feelings, sensations, thoughts and behaviours fall within this description, including:

➤ feelings of numbness, sadness, anger, guilt, anxiety, despair, loneliness, powerlessness, yearning, freedom, relief

➤ physical sensations of shock, fatigue, hollow stomach, aching limbs, dry mouth, breathlessness, tightness in the throat and chest, sensitivity to noise

➤ thoughts of disbelief, confusion, disorientation, obsessional preoccupation with the deceased, visual and auditory hallucinations

➤ behaviours such as sleep disturbance, lack of appetite, absentmindedness, crying, sighing, restless overactivity, searching, calling out, lethargy, dreams, visiting the grave and special places, treasuring reminders and avoiding reminders.

It is important to note that although the intensity of these reactions can be alarming, both for the bereaved person and to those around, they can all be regarded as appropriate responses. It is often the duration of the response which calls it into question as 'usual'.

Grief reactions in bereaved parents are often seen to be more extreme than in other groups. For example, suicidal thoughts and feelings are common to bereaved parents. It is also quite usual for parents to keep the (child's) room unchanged and the (child's) clothes unwashed for a much longer period than would be considered usual in other bereavements. Too often the intensity and chronic nature of the grief reactions of bereaved parents attract labels such as pathological, abnormal or unhealthy.

The features of grieving for a child thus establish a different set of norms. Does that mean that grieving parents are by definition seen as a subgroup outside the mainstream, as destined to experience problematic grieving, and therefore incapable of achieving a resolution of their grief?

Resolution of grief is a difficult concept for parents. Many would reject the idea that grieving for one's child can ever end, and some consciously choose to stay with the intensity of their early grief as a mark of loyalty to the child they can no longer care for. The saying 'time heals' holds a hollow promise for John, whose 10-year-old daughter Clare died during a heart operation, and who speaks here for a significant proportion of bereaved parents:

> When newcomers join us at the Centre, they remind us all of how we were not so long ago, and for me that's good. I don't ever want to leave that behind. I want to always be reminded of the intensity of what I felt, and time robs you of that.'

The concept of *enduring grief* is one that seems entirely appropriate to parents whose prime task is to keep alive the memory and meaning of their child's life. Marking anniversaries, birthdays and holding a picture of the child's would-have-been development, are ways of continuing a lifelong duty of care.

Peppers and Knapp (1980) coined the phrase 'shadow grief' to describe the burden of grief that mothers of children who died in infancy carry for the rest of their lives. The shadow may cast a black pall at significant times, but is always in the background as an aching reminder of the qualified joy of giving life. For some, this 'shadow grief' may recede with time, but for most parents this sense of enduring sorrow is both natural and normal.

This concept of ongoing grief can be compared to the grief experienced by parents of children with long-term disabilities, which Susan Roos describes as 'chronic sorrow' (Roos, 2002). She writes with the authority of a parent of one daughter who has died and another who is severely disabled. This is her definition of chronic loss, a concept first developed by Olshansky (1962):

> 'A set of pervasive, profound, continuing, and recurring grief responses resulting from significant loss or absence of crucial aspects of oneself (self-loss) or another living person (other-loss) to whom there is a deep attachment. The way in which the loss is perceived determines the existence of chronic sorrow. The essence of chronic sorrow is a painful discrepancy between what is perceived as reality and what continues to be dreamed of. The loss is ongoing since the source of the loss continues to be present. The loss is a living loss.' (Roos, 2002, p. 26)

While Roos applies this definition mainly to living with disability, she concedes that the parent whose child has died may continue to grieve for what might have been.

Clearly, the conventional theories that look towards the resolution of grief are inadequate when applied to the death of a child.

The Compassionate Friends (TCF), the self-help organisation for bereaved parents, have developed a language that translates bereavement theory according to their own experience of the bereavement journey. Within TCF's own terms of reference, the course of grief is defined as follows:

➤ *Newly bereaved.* This stage represents the tension between reality of loss and a sense of a future together despite the separation. Linking objects may capture this tension, such as treasured toys, clothes and photographs. Socially, parents will hope that family and friends will not expect them to snap out of their grief after weeks or months.

➤ *Into their grief.* Identity seems to be an important issue at this stage, as parents have to reassess their relation to work and family life. Marriages may experience conflict as both partners seek to find their own best ways of coping with overwhelming feelings. Or perhaps one parent will associate with one aspect of the child, while the other parent holds another aspect. Socially, for members of TCF, shared understanding can lead to more confident communication of needs to the wider community.

➤ *Well along in their grief.* Here the tension is between letting go and holding on. The tension may be to do with feelings such as guilt or anger, or it may relate directly to the image of the child and what that image means. Memories move with the present. Socially, the meaning of present and future is connected to one's identity as a bereaved parent.

➤ *Resolved as much as it will be.* Grief does not abate, but it changes.

Looking back, there is a sense of difference. The transformation of the inner bonds with the dead child is complex but eventually, hopefully, can be part of ongoing life, helping to make meaning rather than destroy it. Socially, there may be a desire to make sense of this pain, to work for others' benefit, to make a difference. In TCF, as well as in the wider community, parents can find a developing bond with their child through new developments in their own lives – as a parent to a new child, as a fundraiser or a befriender.

NEW UNDERSTANDINGS OF GRIEF

During the 1990s the field of bereavement theory was illuminated by a multidisciplinary, international group of researchers who were said to represent a postmodernist view of grief. Writers such as Margaret and Wolfgang Stroebe from Holland, Mary and Kenneth Gergen, Robert Hansson, Dennis Klass, Phyllis Silverman, and Steven Nickman from the USA and Simon Rubin from Israel, challenged the dominant twentieth century models as needing expansion and revision. These challenges are particularly helpful for our understanding of parental grief.

In 1992 Stroebe, *et al.* published a ground-breaking article entitled *Broken hearts or broken bonds* which questioned the prevailing view that good adjustment to bereavement is seen as the breaking of ties between the bereaved and the deceased. They pointed out that historically this was not always so, as reflected in nineteenth-century English literature. The more romantic notion of love and death in Victorian times viewed the breaking of bonds as destroying identity and the meaning of life.

Twentieth-century psychology, by contrast, encouraged goal orientated behaviour, and valued efficiency, rationality, independence and autonomy.

Applied to grief, debilitating responses were seen as problematical until worked through to the restoration of normal functioning. The idea of 'letting go' was commonly seen as desirable and necessary for building a new identity. Consequently the principles of grief counselling followed the view that the bereaved person had to be helped to give up their attachment to the dead; or conversely, those who persist in retaining bonds with the dead were seen as in need of counselling.

If bereavement theory is subject to historical perspective in the Western world, it is further challenged by a comparison with grief in other cultures. Japanese rituals, for example, encourage continued contact with the deceased. The placing of food on the altar dedicated to a loved one is regarded as normal practice in Japan. This provides an interesting comparison with the buying of a birthday cake for a dead child and how that would be viewed in the West.

Stroebe, *et al.* concluded their article published in the *American Psychologist*, October 1992, by arguing for:

> '. . . an appreciative understanding of grief in all its varieties . . . that there are many goals that can be set, many ways to feel, and no set series of stages

... that many forms of expression and behavioural patterns are acceptable reactions to loss.'

(Stroebe, *et al.*, 1992, p. 1211)

Continuing bonds

By 1996 Klass, Silverman and Nickman continue and strengthen the argument for respecting the importance of *continuing bonds* in their introduction to the book carrying these words as the title. They point out that the prevailing twentieth-century models of grief not only contained cultural assumptions that valued disengagement as the goal of mourning, but they also overlooked some important evidence to make the theory fit. This took the form of research findings about the experience of surviving spouses having an ongoing sense of the dead partner, which was seen as a denial of the reality of the loss.

Changes in fostering and adoption practices are also quoted as challenging the conventional view that it is not possible to be involved with more than one attachment at a time. Klass, Silverman and Nickman point out:

'To insist on a separateness that keeps very clear boundaries between people requires a view of human functioning that fails to appreciate the importance of connection and relationship.'

(Klass, Silverman and Nickman, 1996, p. 15)

They argue that an ongoing sense of relationship is both natural and normative. An inner representation of the dead person replaces the living reality without denying the loss. The task of relocating the deceased, as described by Worden, is about accommodating a relationship which is different and which changes over time. The other contributors to *Continuing Bonds* consider different aspects of bereavement but have a consistent message for the reader:

'. . . that the resolution of grief involves continuing bonds that survivors maintain with the deceased and that these continuing bonds can be a healthy part of the survivor's ongoing life. Now the challenge for those who support the bereaved is about how to help them hold and adapt the continuing relationship in a new way, rather than to separate from it.'

(Klass, Silverman and Nickman, 1996, p. 22)

These shifting perspectives generally offer a more flexible and positive understanding of parental experience of enduring grief. The fact that *the death of a child is forever* (the title of Rubin's chapter in *Handbook of Bereavement*, Stroebe, Stroebe and Hansson, 1993) is validated.

Rubin directs our attention to how continuing bonds can be respected and accommodated in a way that minimises any damaging effects on the family as a result of the child's death.

When the reality of the continuing relationship between parent and child beyond the grave is recognised socially, the parent is better able to adapt to the internalised representation of the child. They can grow and age together.

> 'The end of grief is not severing the bond with the dead child, but integrating the child into the parent's life and into the parent's social networks in a different way than when the child was alive.'
>
> (Klass, Silverman and Nickman, 1996, p. 199)

Effective social support is therefore crucial to how bereaved parents can cope and live with their loss.

Dual process model of grief

While traditional models have focused primarily on the painful emotions of loss, this model – developed by Stroebe and Schut (1999) – recognises that there is another process at work for the grieving person, which is about avoiding the feelings and getting on with daily living. Similarly Martin and Doka (2000) talk about intuitive grievers, who focus on the pain of the loss, and instrumental grievers, whose way of coping focuses on activity. The two processes of loss and restoration are seen as equally valid and necessary, and that most people will naturally oscillate between them. This new perspective recognises that individual responses to grief are naturally varied and reflect the social/cultural expectations. Perhaps this dual process can be seen more readily in the conventional gender split in bereaved parents, where stereotypically the mother expresses the intuitive feelings (for both of them) and the father takes on the action-oriented role (for both of them). It has been proposed by Schut, *et al.* (1997) that, in therapy, intuitive grievers are better helped by a balancing cognitive approach, and instrumental grievers better helped by being confronted by their feelings.

Positive grief psychology

The more fluid and flexible understanding of grief in contemporary thinking is reflected in the movement towards recognising the human capacity for growth through adversity. This is not a 'Pollyanna' view of grief, but an understanding of how traumatic experiences can bring opportunities for positive psychological changes. This concept is not new: the idea of personal gain through suffering is to be found in the major religions of Hinduism, Buddhism, Judaism, Christianity and Islam. In the tradition of humanistic psychology, Rogers (1961) and Maslow (1987) emphasised the capacity for becoming fully functioning human beings, always growing towards our full potential. Other significant figures in this trend include Frankl (1959), a holocaust survivor who understood that the search for meaning can transform one's experience of tragedy; Seligman (1998), who rescued psychology from a medical model of illness and treatment and initiated a general shift towards a positive conceptualisation of mental health; Joseph and Linley (2006), who have developed these ideas into a coherent approach to positive therapy; and Yalom (2008), the existential psychotherapist who has encouraged our capacity for finding positive meaning in death.

The essential message of positive grief psychology is that victims can be survivors.

(*See* Chapter 10 for more on Joseph and Linley's concept of 'adversarial growth' and Yalom's notion of 'rippling'.)

Theories of intervention

Attention is now focused on some models which have made a useful contribution to therapeutic interventions when working with bereaved people. These approaches may have grown out of various theoretical understandings of grief but are principally concerned with practical strategies.

Whirlpool of grief

This model of parental experience of grief comes from the work of Dr Richard Wilson, a consultant paediatrician at Kingston Hospital who worked closely with bereaved parents who had lost a child through Sudden Infant Death (SID). Back in the 1980s, he was aware that conventional models of grief with their stages and phases did not sufficiently take into account the experience of families he knew. The alternative model he constructed (Wilson, 1992) has been well received by parents trying to make sense of their experience.

The model depicts an unsuspecting oarsman rowing along the 'River of

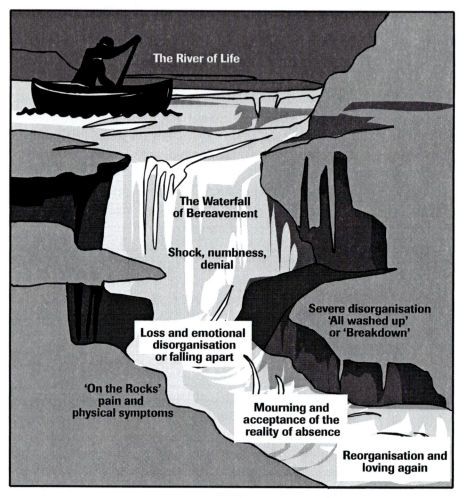

The River of Life

The Waterfall
of Bereavement

Shock, numbness,
denial

Severe disorganisation
'All washed up'
or 'Breakdown'

Loss and emotional
disorganisation
or falling apart

'On the Rocks'
pain and
physical symptoms

Mourning and
acceptance of the
reality of absence

Reorganisation and
loving again

FIGURE 2.1 The whirlpool of grief (Richard Wilson)

Life' who is suddenly plunged down the 'Waterfall of Bereavement' to the 'Whirlpool of Grief' below. The whirlpool carries one round and round, visiting the same emotions time and again, with the occasional respite in the shallows and the risk of being cast against the rocks. The time spent in this period of disorganisation will vary, and some who have been washed up on a bank will choose to stay there. But when the time is right for reorganisation, the 'River of Life' leads away from the whirlpool to calmer waters (*see* Figure 2.1).

Those who have come across this analogy have found it a helpful and attractively simple model. These are Richard Wilson's comments about it:

> 'It may be a little fanciful. However, it is less rigid than suggesting that there are stages of grief which must be completed. People cannot be healed by shepherding them through a fixed treatment plan; however, we may be of some assistance as they make their way along their own difficult and personal journey.
>
> Grief is a turbulent time, and although there may be precious periods of calm, violent emotions which had seemed to be over can return. They are innumerable and all valid. In grief there is a disorganisation of life and thought and values, but most people are then able to reorganise their life in a new way. Although old emotions can always return in almost the same intensity, they do so less frequently and for shorter periods of time.'

The value of this model is that it emphasises the need to listen to parents rather than rely on a taught framework. Bereavement support requires skill and sensitivity rather than knowledge.

Narrative approach

The narrative approach to grief therapy consists of three elements, according to Angus, Levitt and Hardke (1999):

1 telling the story of the loss, what happened and how – described as the *external* narrative
2 describing the impact of the bereavement, how one has been affected – known as the *internal* narrative
3 reflecting on what this loss means to the teller – the *reflexive* narrative.

The ultimate aim of the therapy is to work together towards finding a version of the 'story' that allows for adjustment to the loss. For some, this may be an acceptance of new realities; for others it may involve exploring other ways of understanding, of finding meaning, from their loss. This search for meaning may sound futile to newly bereaved parents, but ultimately they have to find some way of living with their loss. The stories in Chapter 10 are examples of how some bereaved parents have found ways of constructing meaning from their children's lives and deaths which enable them to find new purpose in their own lives.

Compass and map

Machin (2009) has developed a new model for understanding one's grief experience and using that understanding to establish appropriate ways of working. During her long experience of working with bereaved people, she noticed three broadly different reactions within a Range of Responses to Loss (RRL):

1 where the distress from the grief is *overwhelming*
2 where emotions are faced and the consequences are approached with realism – described as a *balanced/resilient* reaction
3 where the need to suppress emotions leads to a very *controlled* reaction.

The RRL model sees the absence of resilience and heightened distress as evidence of vulnerability and uses the identified spectrum of grieving responses as a theoretical compass to help formulate a picture of the nature of individual grief. From this model she has constructed a self-assessment tool, the Adult Attitude to Grief scale, which provides a way of mapping or profiling a client's grief. When the scale is repeated it can show changes taking place over time, and can indicate the various therapeutic interventions that might most appropriately be applied.

> 'For the practitioner, the RRL model provides a structure for appraising the client's grief reaction, and gives a focus to the helping process by indicating the desired direction of change from vulnerability to resilience.'
>
> (Machin, 2009, p. 9)

A systemic approach

Most traditional models have focused on the grief experienced by individuals, whereas family systems theories look at how the loss impacts on the family as a unit. Ways of dealing with the loss will depend on the family's belief systems and values, and family members take on different roles. These systems in turn are shaped by the wider culture to which they belong, which will determine attitudes to death as well as traditional family roles. Family systems and social networks will also dictate what support is acceptable and available.

From this perspective it follows that interventions involving the family may be preferable to working with individuals. Working with the family carries the acceptance that all will be affected, albeit in different ways, and avoids the singling out of one family member who is seen as not coping. Ways of relating to each other and ways of dealing with previous losses can be fruitfully explored. This is where geneograms really come into their own! (*See* Appendix D.) Family members can be helped to find ways of respecting each other's needs and supporting each other appropriately.

Even if it is not appropriate to work with the family, it still makes sense to work with the individual systemically – that is, to see the individual in the context of their family and wider systems of social and cultural settings.

WHAT THE DEATH OF A CHILD MEANS FOR DIFFERENT FAMILY MEMBERS

Parents

As noted above, the grieving of parents may become 'as resolved as much as it will be', but will never be over and done with. Parents suffer multiple losses when their child dies. Obviously the primary loss relates to the attachment and dependency of a unique individual, while the absence of a child represents much more. Parents will also be grieving other losses:

➤ part of their own sense of self, physically, emotionally and spiritually
➤ their connection to the future
➤ unfulfilled expectations and ambitions
➤ some of their own treasured qualities and talents
➤ a source of love and acceptance
➤ a sense of power and control over what happens to them
➤ social status and social contacts.

The loss of a child is perceived as different to other griefs. As one parent put it:

> 'When you lose your parents, you lose your past; when you lose a child, you lose your future.'

The relationship between parents will be tested, and the whole family system will be stressed. For many mothers there is a particular threat to their identity when a child dies. For many fathers, the death of a child is a real assault on their essential role as provider and protector.

Age of the parent

Research seems to indicate that younger parents seem better able to adapt to the loss of a child, while older parents appear to be less capable of recovering from the extreme chaos of the experience (Stroebe, Stroebe and Hansson, 1993).

Age of the child

The age of the child is a principal factor in the significance of the loss, although the death of a child at any age is untimely. A preterm or newborn baby has a fantasy existence for the parents and remains a dream-child in death. A baby who dies within the first year of life leaves the aching arms of a mother from whom he has hardly separated physically. At this age bonding with both parents (or principal carers) is likely to be at its most intense.

As the young child develops, so does its place in the family. Again, a first child will become central to the parents' emotional life. Sometimes a child takes on a special significance for one of the parents: a mother may feel that a particular child 'belongs' to her, or a father may identify strongly with one child as meeting his own needs. As the child becomes more of a real person, developing a separate identity, relationships become more complex. Ambivalent feelings and conflict inevitably affect the child–parent relationship in the teenage years. As one of the tasks of adolescence is to separate from parents and achieve independence, the death of a teenager is likely to leave in its wake a complicated web of unresolved feelings.

Effect on parents

Effects on the individual parent will obviously vary according to the quality of the relationship with the child, personality, previous experience of loss and what kind of support is available. Parents are often affected by doubts of their sanity and their worth.

➤ 'Am I going mad?' is a usual response to the extreme distress and disorganisation of the early months of mourning.
➤ 'Can I go on?' is a usual response to the feelings of worthlessness and despair that make it hard to face another day.
➤ 'I'd like to join him' is a usual response to feelings that the child has deserted the parent, and the parent has failed the child.

The parenting role

Effects on the parenting role will obviously be dramatic when an only child dies. In the eyes of society, they are no longer parents, no longer a family. The direct line of genetic descent has come to an end. Where there are other children, parental grief is likely to be inhibited and tempered by their needs, which may cause resentment or relief. When the surviving children are young, or when other pregnancies quickly follow the bereavement, mothers in particular do not have the space and time to themselves to grieve and are vulnerable to depression. On the other hand, parents who find they can think only of the dead child have little interest or energy for their other children. They may be aware of this and feel guilty about it but it takes a huge effort to do otherwise. Women whose entire identity and self-esteem depend on motherhood may lose a vital sense of self, suffer chronic guilt and face a huge task of adjustment.

Fathers who see themselves as the family provider and protector will feel they have failed in their responsibility, and this may threaten their sense of manhood.

The marriage or partnership

Effects on the marriage or partnership will depend largely on the strength of the couple's relationship beforehand. Any needs that are not being met will be magnified by the loss and cause resentment, particularly if the child supplied some of those needs for one or other of the parents. Initially, a reasonably open and trusting relationship will allow the parents to comfort each other, although, as time goes on, even the closest of couples find that grief separates them in some way – it is essentially a lonely experience. Two people cannot grieve at the same pace nor tend to each other's needs without sacrificing their own. One father put it this way: 'It's like both of you having flu at the same time. You feel so wretched that you can't help your partner.'

Another major factor is the different ways in which the partners may express their grief. Stereotypically, the mother copes with her pain by crying and talking, while the father copes by being active and busy. These differences may be respected, but are more likely to cause resentment that the husband does not appear to be grieving or that the wife is draining him emotionally. They may turn to others for understanding and thus widen the rift. However it happens, a significant number of bereaved couples end up living separately, and most couples experience severe strains on their relationship.

Dot, whose only child Christine died from cystic fibrosis, reflects here on how she and her husband grew apart after Christine's death:

'Bob and I started by grieving together, but after those first two weeks in the depths of despair we couldn't keep in step. I'd look across at him and think, "He's not thinking about Christine at this moment, and so if I say something now, I will be invading his peace . . . let him have this break". But then as time went on, I realised that I could cope with my own very mixed emotions. In a way I was happier not to have to share them. I suppose in my own way I was shutting other people out, including Bob, but somehow that felt safer to me. I think that was the trigger point for grieving apart. Bob then threw himself into his work, and I was left to pick up the pieces of my life, and so our different ways of coping took us further apart. I think grief is such an individual thing that I don't believe you can grieve as a couple.'

John and Sue, whose second child David died of cancer, also found that they grieved in separate ways, but found a way of communicating their needs, which strengthened their relationship. John explains:

'A major factor which helped to bind us together was our relationship with our daughter, Jane. Answering the questions of a three-year-old forced us to bring things out in the open for ourselves.'

Grandparents

Grandparents have an acute sense of broken continuity in the fabric of their own family as well as grieving the loss of the individual child. The effects of losing a grandchild are often underestimated.

The two-generation gap can free grandparents to indulge the child with the kind of attention and affection that creates a special bond between them. Grandchildren represent a continuing link with the future at a time of life when one is increasingly aware of one's own mortality. Grandparenting presents another opportunity to endow children with hopes and expectations, although often tempered by a more realistic view and more tolerant attitudes.

Some grandparents will have been involved directly with the care of the child, particularly when both parents are in employment outside the home or when a young mother is still living at home. In these cases the grandparent takes on a parenting role and the intensity of grief is more akin to that of the parent. Grandparents are also likely to be closely involved with the support of both child and parents in the case of terminal illness.

It is this dual role and relationship that causes most anguish to grandparents. They suffer their own grief, and are affected deeply by their own child's grief. They often feel helpless and inadequate in the support they can offer, frustrated by their inability to comfort and protect. This was Diane's experience:

> 'Other people feel I shouldn't be grieving the way I am, because Anthony was only a grandson. We weren't just nanna and grandson, we were friends. In my case, I'm grieving not only for Anthony, but for my daughter as well. I found I couldn't help her.'

Siblings

Brothers and sisters have been called 'the forgotten mourners'. Sadly, their own grief reactions are often overlooked. Older siblings may be encouraged to 'be strong' for their parents. The effects of sibling loss on young children are not easily remembered or understood, and their needs are not always expressed directly. The age and developmental stage of the grieving child is an important factor, of course, but before looking at different age groups, what are the common factors affecting all siblings?

First, there is the parents' grief and the ways in which their reactions affect their other children. What happens at the time of the death and what the surviving children are told are both crucially important. At any age, a child will be affected by the parent's distress and made anxious by upheaval in the home and family. There is a natural inclination to protect children from witnessing their parents' grief. Yet it is essential for them to see their parents mourn, or they will believe that the dead child was not loved and fear that they would not be mourned either if they were to die.

Siblings are also affected by the impact on the family as a system and the balance of relationships within it. All are required to adjust to the void left by the dead child. One consequence may be that a surviving sibling 'takes the place' of the dead child, fulfilling a particular role with regard to one or both of the parents. Another possible outcome, in a situation where the dead child was intensely idealised by the parents, is that a sibling can become the scapegoat for parental anger and guilt. She finds herself competing with an angel, and is found wanting. Families that normally function by sharing feelings and being open about difficulties will obviously fare better than those that avoid emotions. Families that already have disordered patterns and a history of conflict may be plunged into chaos by the traumatic loss of a child, with serious consequences for all family members.

At any age, siblings lose an ally, particularly when left as an only child. Sibling relationships tend to be ambivalent, with love and affection interwoven with resentment and rivalry. Whatever that balance, the sibling loses a playmate or companion, and someone to identify with in the generation struggle with the adult world. For twins and siblings of a similar age the natural bond is closer. Older siblings are likely to be left with feelings of responsibility and maybe irrational guilt that they could not protect their younger brother or sister. Younger siblings are left with a feeling of insecurity following the failure of their older brother or sister to pave the way to adulthood successfully.

Ages and stages

The age of the sibling is seen as the key factor in anticipating the child's experience of grief, and so provides guidance as to what to say and do. Often, the adults involved will be wary of exposing a young child to information or experiences that she is assumed to be 'too young to understand'. Before going on to describe the features relevant to age groups, it is important to note that children do not automatically reach a new level of understanding on a birthday! Children mature at different rates, and any significant loss may cause regression to a previous stage of development: for example, an eight-year-old will cling to mother again like a four-year-old. It is also helpful to remember that knowledge comes through experience: what a child understands depends more on her previous experience of the world than on her age.

A word of caution about how adults perceive children, because the way we communicate our understanding is determined by the level of language we use. Children are exposed to images of death, via the media and religious symbolism, long before they have the words to describe them. Therefore the tendency is always to underestimate what a child can understand. At the same time, a child's emotional immaturity restricts the ability to cope with intense distress for long periods. This leads to the tendency to underestimate the effects of the bereavement. (*See* Chapter 6 pp 125–7, *Guidelines for talking with children*, for more on ages and stages.)

Most common anxieties for siblings

Across the board, the most common anxieties of siblings can be crudely summarised as:

➤ 'Did I cause it?'
➤ 'Will I die too?'
➤ 'Who now cares for me?'

It follows that key needs for siblings are information, reassurance and attention. It is important to remember that the complex effects of the *secondary losses* experienced by siblings, such as the loss of normality and parental attention, can be more traumatic than the bereavement itself.

Concept of enduring grief for siblings

Karen's sister died suddenly when she was 10 and Karen was six years old. As an adult, Karen continues to miss Elaine at a deep level:

> 'All the important events in my life that have taken place have never been complete because there is always someone missing. My wedding was difficult for me as Elaine would have been my bridesmaid and totally involved in the preparations. Then there have been the births of my two children – I had no big sister to share these wonderful moments with. It just seems to get harder and harder as time goes by. I also struggle with my emotions if my children are ill, though I put a brave face on to everyone. I live in constant fear that they will be taken away from me, and I know this fear will never leave me until I go to my grave.'

What helps?

The following are commonly identified as being helpful to siblings, with the benefit of hindsight:

➤ being told what was happening
➤ being involved, especially going to the funeral
➤ thinking and talking about the loss
➤ meeting other children who have lost a brother or sister
➤ talking to someone outside the family – someone who shows care and understanding without being intrusive.

This last point is illustrated by Rebecca, who was 19 when her sister Anna died suddenly, aged 15:

'I really did appreciate the concern shown by my college chaplain. He cared about me as a grieving individual, rather than about my parents or my dead sister . . . whereas it did feel like friends and family were much more concerned about my parents than about me.'

What makes things worse?

Again, with hindsight, the following are commonly reported as making things harder for the grieving sibling:

➤ being sent away at the time of the death
➤ being excluded from the funeral
➤ being left out of decisions
➤ other children saying hurtful things
➤ not being able to concentrate at school or college
➤ telling other people who don't know what to say.

MOURNING RITUALS

Some features particular to the death of a child affect the bereavement and mourning rituals. These may be practical differences related to the age of the child, cultural differences related to the status of the child or differences of emphasis to do with the special relationship between parent and child.

Given the enduring nature of parental grief, strongly marked by feelings of failure and guilt, it is very important to parents that they 'do their best' for their child after death, which is one aspect of bereavement rituals. For themselves, and for others too, rituals also help to make the loss real and aid the mourning task of learning to live without the presence of the loved one. A third function of rituals is to provide social recognition of the death and public expression of the emotions aroused.

At the time of death

Most religious faiths have rites that are performed with the aid of a priest, minister or holy person, to prepare the dying for the life to come and to lay the dead to rest. Common to those of all faiths, and those with none, is the need to say goodbye to the child, which is in itself a ritual. Seeing, touching, holding and talking to the child all have added significance when the death was unexpected and sudden, and in the case of perinatal death involves saying hello as well as goodbye.

Not all believers in a particular religion keep the same observance of traditional rituals, although it is important to be aware of orthodox practice. For example, distress may be caused to both the Muslim and Hindu family if a child's body is touched after death by a non-believer, although disposable gloves may be used if the family are unable to prepare the body themselves. Removing a lock of hair would be offensive to Muslims, and strict adherents of Islam may discipline themselves to show no emotion at the death of their child, believing it to be the will of Allah. For an orthodox Jewish child, the first acts of shutting the eyes, binding up the jaw and laying the arms straight are traditionally done by a family member. Good practice in hospitals includes known protocols about what to do and who to consult regarding various cultural and religious practices.

The legal ritual of registering the death, and the practical task of informing friends, family and officialdom that the child has died, are ways in which the reality of bereavement is faced and rehearsed.

The absence of formal rituals such as registration is much regretted by those whose baby died before the legal age of viability. It is so important for the family to have something to show that this baby had a life.

Funeral rites

The placing of mementoes, such as a favourite toy in the coffin or on the grave is a powerful symbol of the continuing link between parent and child beyond the grave. In different forms this practice has a universal application. The following is an observation of an American Indian custom:

> 'Both among the Ojibway and other Indian tribes it is a very general custom to cut off a lock of hair in remembrance of their deceased children, especially those still at the breast, and wrap it up in paper and gay ribbons. Round it they lay the playthings, amulets and clothes of the little departed. These form a tolerably long and thick parcel, which is fastened up crosswise with strings, and can be carried like a doll. They give this doll a name signifying "misery" or "misfortune", and which may be translated "the doll of sorrow". This lifeless object takes the place of the deceased child. The mourning mother carries it about for a whole year . . . until the spirit of the child has grown sufficiently to be able to help itself along.'
>
> (Kohl, 1985)

Participation in the funeral rites is important to all those who are significantly affected by the death. The question of whether young children should attend the funeral is for the parents to decide and will be considered in more detail in Chapter 5. Those who do not attend can participate in other ways, for example by being involved in decision making about the form of service, choice of music and so on.

In normal circumstances, Jewish and Muslim funerals take place within 24 hours of the death, and Hindus prefer the funeral to take place as soon as possible. If delay is unavoidable, the reasons need to be carefully explained. Coroners' officers will make special arrangements if a post-mortem is required, so that the funeral is not unduly delayed.

After the funeral

Of all the major religions, Islam upholds the most exacting mourning rituals. The family stays at home for the first three days, and food is brought in by relatives. Strict mourning lasts for 40 days, after which the grave is visited on Fridays. Traditional Hindu mourning is a communal affair, with constant visiting of extended family and neighbours. During the first 12 days after the funeral, ritualistic mourning takes place in the family home, led by an experienced female relative, to encourage the open expression of grief.

Having a place to visit, whether it be a grave or garden of remembrance, provides a continuing ritual for the expression of grief. The intense yearning to be physically close to the child again can be so great as to endanger fantasies of digging up the coffin. Initially, life may only be bearable if sustained by daily visits to the grave to reassure the child of continuing love and care. Later, the placing of the headstone is another formal ritual to mark the permanence of death.

Keeping the child's name and memory alive is a primary concern for parents, and at least a temporary concern for others too. Memorial ceremonies provide an opportunity for the child's school to celebrate the child's life and mourn his loss. Family, school and the local community may choose a form of commemoration, such as an award or dedication, or may embark on fundraising activities to benefit an organisation or area of research associated with the child.

Photographs and other mementoes may be avoided initially but eventually treasured. Sorting through the child's possessions is a painful business and may be long delayed. The distribution of mementoes in the form of toys and clothes among family and friends is usually much appreciated, as these are transitional objects linking the past to the future. Sadly, in the case of sudden death, there may be a superstitious reluctance for friends to accept anything belonging to the child.

Clearing the child's room is another important milestone and not one to be hurried. The choice of when it feels right to do this is an individual one and should be left entirely to the immediate family.

Anniversaries and significant times present opportunities to take stock of the journey through grief and to remember the child in a special way. Continuing rituals of birthday cards and birthday cakes are perfectly natural ways of marking 'would-have-been' milestones, and the buying of Christmas presents may be an important way of including the dead child within the living family at a special time. Those who question such a practice as ghoulish or unrealistic need only ask, does it help, or does it hinder, this parent or family?

Inscriptions in a Book of Remembrance are particularly valued by those who have few tangible reminders. Similarly, a joint memorial service, such as the Candle Service held annually in many of our major cities, when a candle is lit for every named child, is another way of using ritual to celebrate life as well as to mourn death.

References

Angus L, Levitt H, Hardke K. Narrative processes in psychotherapeutic change. *J Clin Psychol.* 1999; 55: 1255–70.

Bowlby J. *Attachment and Loss,* Vols 1–3. *Attachment,* Vol. 1, 1969; *Separation: anxiety and anger,* Vol. 2, 1973; *Loss: sadness and depression,* Vol. 3, 1980. New York: Basic Books; 1969–80.

Frankl V. *Man's Search for Meaning.* Boston: Beacon Press; 1959.

Freud S. (1961 – originally published 1917) Mourning and melancholia. In: Strachey J, editor and translator. *The Standard Edition of the Complete Psychological Works of Sigmund Freud.* London: Hogarth Press; Vol. 14, 1961; pp. 243–58.

Joseph S, Linley PA. *Positive Therapy. A meta-theory for positive psychological practice.* London: Routledge; 2006.

Klass D, Silverman P, Nickman S, editors. *Continuing Bonds: new understandings of grief.* London: Taylor & Francis; 1996.

Kohl J. *Kitchi-Gami.* St Paul: Minnesota Historical Society Press; 1985.

Machin L. *Working with Loss and Grief.* Thousand Oaks, CA: Sage Publications; 2009.

Martin TL, Doka KL. *Men Don't Cry . . . Women Do.* Philadelphia: Brunner/Mazel; 2000.

Maslow AH. *Motivation and Personality.* New York: Harper & Row; 1987.

Olshansky S. Chronic sorrow: a response to having a mentally deficient child. *J Soc Casework*. 1962; 43: 191–3.

Parkes CM. *Bereavement: studies of grief in adult life*. New York: International Universities Press/Pelican; 1972.

Parkes CM, Brown RJ. Health after bereavement: a controlled study of young Boston widows and widowers. *Psychosom Med*. 1972; **34**(5): 449–61.

Peppers LG, Knapp RJ. *Motherhood and Mourning*. New York: Praeger; 1980.

Rogers C. *On Becoming a Person*. London: Constable; 1961.

Roos S. *Chronic Sorrow: a living loss*. New York: Brunner-Routledge; 2002.

Schut H, Stroebe M, de Keijser J, *et al*. Intervention for the bereaved: gender differences in the efficacy of two counselling programmes. *Br J Clin Psychol*. 1997; **36**: 63–72.

Seligman MEP. Building human strength: psychology's forgotten mission. *APA Monitor*. 1998; **29**(1).

Stroebe M, Gergen MM, Gergen KJ, *et al*. Broken hearts or broken bonds. *Am Psychol*. 1992; **47**(10): 1205–12.

Stroebe M, Schut H. The dual process model of coping with bereavement: rationale and description. *Death Stud*. 1999; **23**: 197–224.

Stroebe M, Stroebe W, Hansson R, editors. *Handbook of Bereavement: theory, research and intervention*. Cambridge: Cambridge University Press; 1993.

Wilson R. Lecture handout from Child and Death International Conference, Edinburgh 1992.

Worden WJ. *Grief Counselling and Grief Therapy*. 4th ed. London: Routledge; 2008.

Yalom I. *Staring at the Sun: overcoming the dread of death*. London: Piatkus; 2008.

Further reading

Dallos R, Draper R. *An Introduction to Family Therapy: systemic theory and practice*. 2nd ed. Paris: Lavoisier; 2005.

Nixon J, Pearn J. Emotional sequelae of parents and sibs following the drowning or near drowning of a child. *Aust NZ J Psychiatry*. 1977; **11**: 265–8.

Parkinson F. *Post-trauma Stress*. London: Sheldon Press; 1993.

SECTION 2

Good practice guidelines

CHAPTER 3

Professional roles

'Grief wounds more deeply in solitude; tears are less
bitter when mingled with others' tears.'

Seneca's *Agamemnon*

Attention is now focused on the roles and functions of various groups
according to job title. Some, such as the paediatric intensive care nurse or
funeral director, have an essential role to play and will encounter the death
of a child as part and parcel of their work. Others, such as the registrar of
births, marriages and deaths, will have a single and functional contact with
many bereaved families, while health visitors and social workers are likely to
be involved in ongoing support. GPs and spiritual leaders may fill a key supportive role, although only occasionally over a lifetime career. Paramedics
and police personnel are in the front line in emergency situations, and their
initial reactions can do much to help or hinder parents. Teachers seldom
deal with the death of a child, but they too can perform significant functions
and be profoundly affected.

Whatever the level of involvement, this chapter will give information,
reassurance and confidence. Points of likely involvement with the terminally
ill child or bereaved family will be identified and linked to the possible tasks
to be undertaken. Examples of good practice will be illustrated by drawing
on the experience of families and individual professionals.

Different professions are considered alphabetically. If this chapter is
being used for reference, the reader's attention is drawn to the general principles, which apply to everyone, in Chapter 4. In particular it is important
to note the opening lines: *We do not have to be experts to support people with*

their grief. What we can all do to help is assess their needs and our abilities to provide what they need.

BEREAVEMENT SUPPORT WORKERS
Involvement

As a result of a Department of Health report in 2005, all hospitals are required to have a coordinated bereavement support or bereavement care service. A worker in this service will be involved with the parents or family at the time of the death and will facilitate the tasks of the first hours and days following the death. One worker described her meeting with the parents on the ward thus:

> 'The named nurse introduces me to the parents. Then I introduce myself to the (dead) child. I say, "Hi there Johnny. Your parents have been looking after you for so long, and now I am going to look after them for the next couple of days". This is my way of accepting the child and the situation.'

Function

At a time of shock and distress for the parents, the bereavement support worker provides a reassuring presence by explaining what happens next in terms of choices and procedures. Some parents may opt to take the child's body home immediately, perhaps for spiritual or cultural reasons, though more usually the child will be placed in the hospital's bereavement suite in the mortuary until collection by the funeral director or until the post-mortem if required. Babies may be carried from the ward to the bereavement suite by the parents themselves, while an older child will be taken by portering services while the support worker accompanies the parents. The bereavement suite should provide a comfortable and peaceful environment for viewing, touching and holding the child by the parents and family members, who may come from far afield. The parents themselves are often exhausted at this stage and the support worker can reassure them of help with practical tasks such as registering the death once they have returned home for some rest. The support worker can book the time to visit the registrar and accompany the parents, and later facilitate the release of the child's body to the funeral director.

Concerns

Dealing with a large number of family members visiting the bereavement suite at the same time can be stressful, especially if some relatives are giving vent to anger. The bereavement support worker's first priority is to support the parents, and they may be involved in reminding concerned grandparents how important it is not to take away control and choices from the parents – such as planning the funeral for them.

Encouraging the parents to leave the child in order to get some rest can be tricky and then witnessing the parents leaving their dead child in the bereavement support worker's care is a powerful and challenging moment.

A situation which may need careful handling is when the child is brought in from the community and there is other agency involvement following a sudden and unexpected death in infancy (SUDI), RTA, or suspected non-accidental injury.

Good practice

The cardinal guideline for the bereavement support worker is to facilitate choices to empower parents who have lost control over their child's life.

Being alongside parents at such an emotional time requires honesty, sensitivity, and genuineness. Good communication skills are paramount, in giving good information, keeping an open dialogue going with the parents, and in choosing one's language carefully. An awareness of ethical issues is essential, particularly in being clear about confidentiality boundaries.

In terms of self-care, taking time for emotional recovery once the parents and family have left the bereavement suite is important, and clinical supervision should be available.

CHAPLAINS/SPIRITUAL CARE ADVISORS
Involvement

Typically a paediatric hospital has had chaplains from principal denominations of the Christian church, with access to spiritual leaders from other faiths. In this age of respecting difference and diversity, hospitals are now moving towards establishing multi-faith teams of spiritual care advisors.

A chaplain or spiritual care advisor may be involved at the time of the death, or over months or even years prior to the death, as the child's illness progresses or further surgery is required. Daily ward visiting provides the opportunity to make initial contact, and thereafter to express ongoing empathy and concern.

As death approaches, prayers, blessings and other rituals are performed for those parents who request them. After death the chaplain may be a natural choice to help plan and conduct the funeral service, with later visits at significant times.

Function

'We do so little – and they perceive it as so much', one chaplain comments. But when she adds, 'What I do is journeying with parents, walking alongside them in their darkest hours', it is obvious why her work is appreciated.

As stated above, the spiritual care advisor has specific roles to play at significant times, but more generally the ongoing availability and comforting presence are key. Absorbing concerns and anxieties may lead to a mediating role, to aid communication with medical personnel.

The chaplain is also available to hospital staff for spiritual advice and support.

Concerns

I asked one chaplain what challenges she faced in her job, and she replied, 'Sometimes God is challenged'. She went on to explain that anger with God is a natural response from parents, and that response requires understanding rather than defensive explanations or statements of faith.

It seems natural that one's personal faith will be tested by the anguish caused by the untimely death of a child.

Good practice

Respect for others at their most vulnerable demands taking account of the parents' own faith stance to determine what spiritual support they want. Meeting people where they are and 'walking alongside them' is about responding to their spiritual needs rather than imposing one's own beliefs.

Being respectful, empathic and genuine are the core conditions of any helping relationship, and spiritual advisors are probably expected to demonstrate these attitudes in all that they do. Living up to such expectations requires enormous commitment.

Being genuine means avoiding the kind of platitudes that in the past have been associated with some pious and paternalistic faith leaders. Such assurances as 'God only takes the best' may seek to comfort but are motivated by helplessness. One needs to be able to tolerate such feelings to do this job well.

Good practice includes self-care, and the chaplain needs a support system within the hospital as well as externally through spiritual guidance and supervision.

CLERGY
Involvement
Many families that give little or no active support to their church will fall back on the traditional beliefs and rituals of their culture.

Thus the leader of the local religious community, whether priest, minister, imam or rabbi, is nearly always involved at the time of the death or soon after. Hospital chaplains or spiritual care advisors are often involved before the death of a terminally ill child, building up supportive relationships with both families and staff (*see* previous entry).

Most clergy offer their pastoral support by visiting the family as soon as they hear of the death of a child in their area, often from the undertaker, and continue to visit for as long as the family wish. The priest or minister who has an accumulated knowledge of the family history is ideally placed to receive the expression of grief.

However, now that fewer than one in four babies is baptised into the Church of England, the reality is that the spiritual meaning of the church is no longer relevant to the majority.

Function
Unless the family already has an allegiance to a particular church, the parochial role is restricted to conducting the funeral service.

John, an Anglican priest in a town parish, describes himself as a 'necessary functionary' for death rituals in a secular society. He makes a point of visiting the family as soon as possible, 'just to listen and act as a buffer for the injustice and anger they feel'. He has learned that there is nothing he can say in answer to the question. 'Why has God done this to my innocent child?' except to acknowledge the distress. Later, perhaps, is the time for engaging with the family in a spiritual search for meaning, but for now he resists the platitudes of false comfort. Practically speaking, he can advise the family of their options and funeral arrangements, and help them to make informed choices. Parish clergy are in a good position to slow down well-meaning relatives who rush parents into hasty decisions.

Concerns

As the traditional role of the established church becomes eroded, there are increasing dilemmas posed by the trend towards essentially humanist funerals. Family requests for the inclusion of popular music and secular readings may be seen as undermining the religious significance of the funeral service. Clergy are as subject to stress as anyone in the face of tragedy and may feel more exposed than most to the extent of human suffering. 'I try not to get over-involved', one priest said, 'but the pathos of some cases just gets to me . . .' Not all clergy are supported by an understanding spouse or fellow priest.

Confidentiality is an important issue, particularly for hospital chaplains, and may add to the stresses.

Good practice

David and Glenda were plunged into a nightmare when their three-year-old daughter, Stacey, suffered unsuspected heart problems during a minor nose operation and died after some hours in intensive care. The Catholic chaplain who was called to give a last blessing to Stacey stayed to comfort the shocked and angry parents and later took them home in his car. Glenda recalls:

> 'He was really good with Dave, who kept on at him about God letting Stacey die. He seemed to understand, and said we had every right to be angry.'

Clergy who are experienced in this area of grief say that expressions of sympathy need to be carefully chosen. Talking of 'God's will' or 'an angel in heaven' is not helpful. Parents of babies who have not been baptised need reassurance that Christian theology no longer sees this as an exclusion from God's grace. Similarly, parents who blame themselves need reassurance that their child's death is not a punishment.

CORONERS
Involvement

All child deaths must be reported to the coroner by law. If the death is expected and natural, no further action is required legally; if unexpected and the cause is unnatural and/or unknown, the coroner orders a post-mortem to be carried out by a paediatric pathologist, unless the cause of death is so obvious (as in some RTAs) that there is no benefit to be gained. If, as a result of a post-mortem, a natural cause of death is revealed, then the death will be registered in the normal way and the coroner takes no further action. In all other cases the coroner will open an inquest to establish the cause of death and details as to how, when and where the child died.

Function

It will be either the coroner or one of the coroner's officers who will take the first call from a paediatrician or police officer reporting the death. In the case of no further action, the coroner will 'sign off' the pink form required by the registrar. If a post-mortem is required, the parents will be contacted to explain the procedure and the choices open to them about what they want to happen to any tissue that is taken. It can be several months before the pathologist's report is available, so the coroner will open an inquest for identification evidence only, to permit disposal of the body, and then adjourn the inquest to establish causation at a later date.

Concerns

Being in charge of a child death inquest, which is usually charged with emotion, can be very stressful. The coroner is putting the family through the agony of reliving the events and perhaps hearing unpleasant detail in a public forum.

However this process can be cathartic, if the evidence provides reassurance to counter parental feelings of guilt and responsibility.

Good practice

Good practice is all about providing information to the parents as and when required, and making oneself available. Even when no further action is required following the reporting of the death, a talk with the family to check that they have no issues to warrant a post-mortem is a recommendation following the Shipman enquiry. The parents should be kept informed, and prepared before an inquest to ensure there are no nasty surprises. The inquest is best kept as informal as possible, and the family should be encouraged to ask questions, either directly or through a lawyer.

While the coroner carries a huge responsibility to carry out the law, there is an equal responsibility to deal with grieving families with compassion and sensitivity.

COUNSELLORS (*see also* Chapter 7, pp 145–53)
Involvement

Counselling may be sought as a direct consequence of the bereavement, probably within the first year; or the loss of a child may be part of a broader picture when someone presents for counselling at a later stage with other issues, such as marital difficulties or depression. The setting for the counselling may be as a private practitioner; as a health practice or EAP (Employee Assistance Programme) counsellor; within hospital, hospice or bereavement services; as part of pastoral care; or belonging to a specialist area relevant to the death, such as termination, cancer or genetics. Counselling may have been offered to the family during the child's illness, which may enable the bereaved to work through their feelings of loss after the death.

Whether self-presenting or referred, the bereaved person enters into a contract with the counsellor that sets out the terms, frequency and objectives of the counselling. This is particularly important for professionals trained as counsellors who are also known in other roles – as a nurse, social worker or GP – so that the client is clear about which role they are using for the purpose of meeting. Professionals who use counselling skills within their work but who are not trained as counsellors should not, of course, lay claim to the title of counsellor, nor encourage others to regard them as a counsellor.

Function

The counsellor's main function is to provide independent psychological support. Lendrum and Syme in the introduction to *Gift of Tears* (1992) refer to being 'enabled, through the presence of another person, to work through our separate griefs and to lay down some of the burdens we had been carrying.'

Whatever the setting, the counsellor seeks to develop a therapeutic relationship within clear boundaries that will promote trust, safety, space, permission, normalisation, support and challenge. Whatever methods are used, the goal will be to find some way of integrating a sense of self before, during and after the death of the child. The relationship with the counsellor is likely to provide the opportunity to re-work issues of attachment, separation and loss.

For those who are already self-aware, the counsellor's role will be more as companion than guide. Others who are less articulate emotionally may require a more educative role from their counsellor to develop inner resources and perhaps learn new strategies.

Concerns

Typically, these are about the counsellor's ability to cope with raw and chronic grief, and the sense of helplessness that often accompanies bereavement counselling. The death of a child is specially poignant and leaves the counsellor vulnerable to her own real or feared losses, particularly in relation to her own children. For a fulltime counsellor dealing exclusively with bereavement there is a concern that her normality becomes centred on death and grief in a world full of accidents and illness. A counsellor constantly exposed to child death may fear losing the capacity to respect the uniqueness of the client's experience. The following observation is made by a counsellor who is also a bereaved parent herself:

> 'I have heard other counsellors express the view that there is a time limit or "shelf-life" for bereavement counsellors. One counsellor actually admitted to me that she felt it was time to leave her current job because she felt that she had heard so much grief that nothing was unique to *her* any more, and she felt that she was doing her clients a disservice. A pretty brave decision when paid counselling jobs aren't easily obtainable and your salary may be important to your family.'

Good practice

Counsellors need good assessment skills, to take into account how the external circumstances of the bereavement and the internal make-up of the prospective client affect the appropriateness of counselling. The counsellor should take into account her level of training and experience in assessing whether she can meet the client's needs, and if she feels unable to do so, will offer best support by referring on. Supervision can be invaluable for these assessment issues. Adequate supervision is essential at all stages, with access to one's own therapy when needed. (*See* Chapter 4 for more on supervision.)

The counselling contract is a mutual agreement between counsellor and client about the nature and purpose of their work together. Clear contracting, clarity of task and regular reviews are all important to maintain safety, confidence and focus. Particular care needs to be given to endings – uncertain or unplanned endings may compound the client's grief, whereas well-managed endings can help the client to re-work some aspects of the bereavement. Membership of a professional association with a code of ethics and complaints procedure is necessary for safe practice and this information should be made available to the client. There is also an obligation on the counsellor to maintain professional development through reading and ongoing training.

FUNERAL DIRECTORS
Involvement
Although legally there is nothing to stop parents managing the child's funeral themselves, nearly all will engage a funeral director to do this. Contact is usually made within hours of the death. Those firms that offer a free basic service in the event of a child's death tend to take a special pride in this very sensitive part of their work.

Function
In the first interview with the parents, the funeral director or receptionist gives information about options and requires answers to difficult questions. Is a burial or cremation preferred? When is the funeral to be? Where will the child's body lie meanwhile? While always respecting the parents' wishes, the undertaker may offer points of view the parents had not considered: in determining burial or cremation, what happens if they move house in a few years? Many parents do not know what they can and cannot do, and may need encouragement to help to dress the child, to take the child out of the coffin or to have the child at home for a while.

In preparing the body for the coffin, special care is taken to present the baby or child in the most natural and attractive way. Photos, handprints and a piece of hair are usually offered to parents.

Male relatives often wish to carry the coffin themselves, which seems more appropriate when the child is young and the coffin small. If preferred, the funeral director and staff will take responsibility for this and other practical tasks, thus freeing the family to give way to their grief.

Concerns

Keeping the balance between compassion and professional detachment can be difficult. Nothing affects staff so much as the preparation of a young child for the coffin, and they will take enormous trouble to do their best for the family. The first interview with shocked and distraught parents can be very stressful.

Good practice

A funeral director with many years' experience believes the guiding principle should be to involve the family in the funeral preparations as much as possible:

> 'I always try to take my instructions from the parents themselves, and encourage them to see and hold the child as often as they wish. If parents are reluctant to take their baby out of the coffin, I hold the baby myself first, to give them confidence and to show my respect.'

Parents should not be rushed into making hasty decisions about funeral arrangements, and value advice about different options, ranging from a full church service to a simple ceremony in the home. The option of opening a new family grave is an important consideration for parents who eventually wish to be laid to rest in the same place as their child.

GENERAL PRACTITIONERS
Involvement

Typically a doctor in general practice will deal with a child death every few years, usually in the traumatic circumstances of a sudden death by accident, and occasionally as the result of chronic illness. In the latter case, the doctor will have been closely involved with the family over a period of time and perhaps since the child's birth. He may have played a significant part in the family's experience of the diagnosis, treatment and palliative care, particularly if the death occurs at home. In the process he may have formed close relationships with the parents and child. The GP leads a primary care team who may be involved over many years with a family for whom the death of a child has far-reaching implications.

A GP looks back over many years' experience in the same three-doctor practice with these comments:

'With hindsight, it is clear that in the management of the bereaved family, the GP, district nurse, practice nurse, health visitor and counsellor amongst others, all play an important part in helping families through their grieving. The surprising thing to me is how long the process lasts, and the extent to which there can be ramifications throughout the family of the deceased.'

Function

The GP is a primary care provider, a central reference point of all community healthcare, and, as such, has a co-ordinating role. Assessment, treatment and referral are key functions. The GP will be a point of first contact for women who miscarry or seek termination of pregnancy. The GP's help is often sought in going through medical reports following a perinatal death. At the time of bereavement, the GP may be called on to alleviate post-trauma distress, and parents certainly appreciate a home visit at this time, particularly following a cot death. The GP provides medical information and advice. In the early days a mild sedative may be prescribed to help with sleep disturbance. Later, treatment of chronic stress and depression will range from advice to psychiatric referral, but in most cases will include some counselling and/or drugs, depending on the GP's resources and approach to mental health. Measures of healthy grieving are the frequency of visits to the practice centre, the nature of presenting symptoms, and the ability to return to work. As GPs are required to confirm fitness to work, they are in an excellent position to monitor the situation. They also provide continuity for the family and are readily accessible when other supports have fallen away. Record-keeping is an important function for providing this continuity of care, enabling the GP to relate behaviour or symptoms to previous losses.

As well as providing frontline support himself, the GP may refer ongoing mental health concerns to counselling or Community Psychiatric Nursing (CPN) services. In so doing, it is important not to pathologise 'normal' grief reactions.

GPs may find the comments of this GP counsellor of interest:

'It's surprising how many GPs feel uncomfortable with bereavement and often refer clients to me within the first weeks of a death, when all they really need to do is to "normalise" grief reactions. My experience has been that the message conveyed is that counselling is a compulsory part of bereavement, when in fact many people, once they realise that their feelings are normal, cope very well on their own.

The impact on siblings is often unrecognised in that I have heard a teenager being told "be strong for your mum and dad" and another "you've got your whole life ahead of you, stop being silly".

(*See* Chapter 2, pp 43–50, for effects on different family members.)

Concerns

Lack of formal preparation and infrequent incidence of child death mean that the GP will have to call on inner resources. Traditional attitudes in the medical profession make it hard to deal with feelings of helplessness and inadequacy when a child dies. It goes against the grain for some doctors to be as open as parents would like them to be, and many are more comfortable with sharing clinical detail than giving emotional support. Similarly, the traditional independence of doctors makes it hard to seek professional support and advice for themselves. Medical training and hospital work encourage the attitude that a doctor can cope with anything; in general practice a doctor is indeed expected to cope with everything, frequently switching from mundane to emotionally demanding tasks. On a practical level, GPs who are motivated to offer direct support have to guard their time and commitment priorities, both in the surgery and in terms of home visiting.

GPs may be subject to irrational criticism from parents. For example, it is a common pattern that parents change to another doctor after a cot death.

Good practice

In responding to a sudden death for the first time, the GP may welcome the following pointers as being valued by families.

➤ Showing that you care and sharing your feeling is much appreciated by parents.

➤ When presented with a dead child clearly beyond resuscitation, remember the value of parents being with their child *for as long as they wish* before handing over to the coroner.

➤ Families will welcome your reassurance that grieving is a gradual process that cannot be hurried, and that you and your team are available for ongoing support.

➤ In prescribing drugs to alleviate distress, be aware that many parents later regret taking any medication which impedes decision making or dulls emotions to an extreme degree.

➤ Advise parents of likely reactions, both physical and emotional, and reassure them of the normality of such symptoms as aching arms, distressing dreams, hearing the child's voice, loss of appetite and libido, anger and guilt.

➤ Encourage siblings to be involved by informing parents of the possible benefits of brothers and sisters seeing the dead child and attending the funeral.

➤ Explain practicalities, such as the coroner's role, registering the death, funeral options.
(*See also* Chapter 5.)

Finally, these are the comments of a senior partner in a busy inner-city general practice:

> 'We all set ourselves high standards, so we may see a child's death as a personal failure. It is important to acknowledge and deal with these feelings. Our professional defences shouldn't get in the way of letting parents see our anxiety, uncertainty or sadness. Also, as a male GP, I can gently challenge the stereotypical father's need to "be strong". Overall, the most important thing is to be there for the family, not necessarily to do something. *Parents require human contact more than cold professionalism.*'

HEALTH VISITORS
Involvement

Where long-term illness or disability leads to death, the health visitor will already be involved with the family, perhaps liaising with other agencies to provide nursery places for siblings, with benefit officers and with support organisations. She has a pivotal role in the communication protocol that follows childhood death. More districts and trusts are now publishing written procedures to formalise existing systems in which the health visitor is responsible for disseminating information from the hospital to the school, community health services and hospital staff. The health visitor has access to medical records and information about the family, knowledge of the community and local resources.

Involvement is immediate as well as automatic, and contact is made with the family as soon as the health visitor is informed of the death, possibly the same day. If the family is known, it may be appropriate to attend the funeral. Follow-up visits may continue up to the first anniversary, depending on the wishes of the parents.

Function

Immediate support on a practical level may include co-ordinating services, explaining procedures, liaising with the GP and providing medical information. Although health visitors are trained to give advice and help, in this situation they are also required to be active listeners, allowing the family to talk through their feelings. Their unique position in the community can provide excellent opportunities for addressing the needs of siblings, grandparents and the concerns of other families following a sudden death.

Follow-up after hospital visits is offered to parents to go over the medical issues. Advice may be sought about surviving siblings and subsequent children. Mothers who are isolated may need a lot of emotional support, facing the health visitor with the dilemma of whether preventive mental health work is consistent with the role and caseload. The level of continuing support will depend partly on the individual's confidence in counselling skills and access to supervision. Referrals to other agencies for further help may be considered appropriate.

Concerns

In areas where there is no established protocol for health visitor liaison, there is always the anxiety about a loophole in communication. The resulting distress to parents when, say, a routine appointment arrives for the dead child, is deeply embarrassing. In the case of sudden death from SIDS or acute illness, the health visitor may be left with doubts and self blame: was there some sign or symptom that was missed, and were visits frequent enough?

Apprehension at the emotional turmoil of the bereaved family and how one will be affected personally is stressful. In visiting the home alone, the health visitor can take on some of the family's feelings of isolation and may well bear the brunt of parental feelings of guilt and blame, and be faced with very difficult questions with no easy answers.

There may be no support structure or formal supervision to help deal with personal reactions and assess appropriate levels of involvement. Where a need for further help for the family is identified, there may be a lack of local counselling and befriending resources.

Good practice

Detailed guidelines are to be found in leaflets published by the Foundation for the Study of Infant Deaths and the Scottish Cot Death Trust. The following advice is taken from discussions with several experienced professionals from different areas.

➤ Be sensitive to the parents' needs and go at their pace, being supportive without taking over.

➤ Avoid saying anything that implies judgement or criticism of the child's care.

➤ Be prepared to listen; share feelings and memories.

➤ Be there for *all* the family, including siblings and grandparents.

➤ Do not give up visiting for fear of intruding (unless requested to do so); continue telephone contact and remember anniversaries.

➤ Familiarise yourself with procedures in your area regarding hospitals, police, funeral arrangements, social services; and research local and national bereavement resources.

A health visitor provides this recent example of how her clinic supported the young mother of a four-month-old cot death baby:

> 'As a single parent with three other young children, Gwen needed a lot of support. My colleague was frustrated that Gwen was unwilling to do all the things advised for healthy grieving, like visiting the baby in the hospital, dressing him, having a photograph and so on. We talked it through as a team, and suggested to my colleague that there might be other members of the family who could be involved, and in fact two of Gwen's sisters were keen to help dress the baby and sort out the funeral and that's what happened. It was important for the family to be in charge.'

HOSPITAL DOCTORS

Involvement

Doctors may be involved in the casualty department, both at children's hospitals and at general hospitals, where they see the victims of accidents, of self-inflicted injuries and of emergency situations. Another obvious area is the intensive care unit, where, by definition, the illness is critical. Deaths occur more rarely on other hospital wards, such as from terminal pneumonia in a child with a chronic disability, or as the outcome of malignant disease and other lifethreatening conditions. Here the consultant will already be a familiar and important person to the child and family, and may have been involved from the time of diagnosis, when grieving begins for many parents. Bereavement issues are also relevant to doctors involved with neonates, stillbirths and terminations for fetal abnormalities.

Function

As well as being responsible for the medical treatment of disease, doctors are concerned with the overall care of the patient, and for paediatricians the patient equals child *and* family. In the case of terminal illness, the consultant has the task of communicating the diagnosis, of explaining the progression of the condition, and keeping parents informed so that joint decisions can be made about treatment choices. This may include the crucial choice between active treatment and palliative care.

The doctor confirms the death, and if the parents are not present at the time, is likely to be the one to inform them. If the death is sudden, another task is to explain the legal process and possibility of a post-mortem. Explanations are required regarding the circumstances that have caused the death, and at this time parents need to know that they will have the opportunity of subsequent meetings to discuss post-mortem reports, answer questions relating to siblings, future children, genetic implications and future support resources.

Some doctors offer routine home or hospital visits for such meetings. Hospital doctors may be interested in these comments made by an experienced GP:

> 'Anecdotally, both from my patients and from other sources, I still hear of cases where the announcement of death or impending death is handled badly. This is rather sad since I feel, as a profession, we should be managing the situation better.
>
> I think in hospital the junior members of the team should have an opportunity to be present at these contacts with relatives, but the sole responsibility for conveying sympathy to the bereaved and supplying them with additional information should come from the top of the team, and this should be standard practice. It is an insult to relatives and an assault on the emotional integrity of junior hospital doctors to expect them to handle that sort of situation on their own, with no previous experience and little training in this area.'

At the time of death, the doctor needs to ensure that immediate support for the family is available from the social services department, chaplain or other designated staff. In the case of the death of a young infant, other practicalities include the control of pain and lactation and help with sleep.

In all deaths, there is a communication role, to liaise with the GP, health visitor and, in certain circumstances, with the community medicine specialist.

Concerns

Newly qualified doctors may find it hard to deal with young parents and older children because of their similarity in age.

Medical ethics are involved in some issues, such as:

➤ whether and when resuscitation efforts should cease
➤ whether active treatment should give way to palliative care
➤ when life-support systems should be withdrawn
➤ the use of donor organs.

Resources can become an overriding concern. Consultants who wish to improve facilities for the child's family, or introduce policies that allow greater parental involvement, will find themselves arguing against colleagues who see death as a non-medical issue.

Professionalism and personal feelings may be in conflict, causing anxiety about one's ability to handle the situation appropriately. Should feelings be shown, uncertainties admitted? How does one develop the skills and sensitivity needed to talk to bereaved parents? And where does the healer go for healing and support?

Good practice

Parents commonly identify several points relating specifically to hospital doctors.

➤ Even if the consultant was not present at the death, parents appreciated the consultant visiting them to acknowledge the death.
➤ Knowing and using the child's name, and looking the parents straight in the eye, conveyed respect.
➤ Expressing regret and appropriate use of touch conveyed real caring. (*See also* Chapter 5.)

As a consultant paediatrician at Alder Hey Hospital, Liverpool, John Sills offered this advice to junior doctors working in casualty or intensive care:

> 'Basically they should show that they care about what has happened, that they respect the child and the family, and that they are there to answer questions. If the death is relatively non-acute they should keep the parents informed, and should liaise with their senior colleagues about what is happening.'

Richard Wilson gained great respect for his work with bereaved families as a consultant paediatrician at Kingston Hospital. These are his comments:

> 'We cannot make the situation better, but we may make it worse, and we must learn to avoid doing so. But we do care and are moved by events. As professionals we want to help, yet difficulties arise in distinguishing between our emotions and needs and those of the parents. We must acknowledge our personal feelings but not let them overwhelm our professional role. The family has need of our help, but we give it not as experts but almost as passers-by whom they have allowed in. There must be organisation and guidelines, but we should have some understanding of ourselves, for only then can we be of use.
>
> When we meet bereaved parents it is important to recognise the individuality of each situation, to know a little theory, to have tips – which come essentially from parents – on what can and cannot be done, to decide our own role, and in particular develop our ability to listen.'

MORTUARY TECHNICIANS
Involvement

In most cases, the mortuary technician oversees the management of the child's body from leaving the hospital ward until collection by the funeral director after the death has been registered, usually within a day or two. The mortuary department includes appropriately furnished viewing facilities for parents and family members to visit the child. Usually the hospital's bereavement support workers will accompany the parents and help guide them through this difficult time, but if the death occurs over a weekend or the bereavement support staff are occupied with other families, the mortuary technician may be required to step in.

When a post-mortem is needed, the mortuary technician will be closely involved with the child's body before and during the examination, and is responsible for the administrative work which follows.

Functions

The technicians are the only people to move the body within the mortuary. Before a post-mortem, they are responsible for organising X-rays and scans. Assisting the pathologist with the post-mortem examination includes replacing removed organs and reconstructing the body. Afterwards, the body is washed and prepared for collection by the funeral director and subsequent viewings by the family, taking care to cover any incision marks. Usually the parents bring the clothes for dressing the baby or child, but if not, suitable clothes will be provided. Gloves are worn at all times, which is an important reassurance for Muslims who require that only those of their own faith should touch the dead body.

After the post-mortem, the inevitable paperwork includes collecting notes for the report and sending off samples to the laboratories.

Concerns

For obvious reasons, RTA deaths and police cases are more challenging to deal with. Arguably, the mortuary technician's job in a children's hospital is not suitable for someone who is a parent of young children, as it would be extremely difficult to completely disconnect emotionally.

One technician commented that the most difficult experiences for her have been when she has also met and talked with the parents, though generally she is not affected emotionally by her work. By contrast, she says:

> 'I couldn't be a nurse. I would find it too hard to cope with sick children. But nothing worse can happen to the child once he or she is dead. The child doesn't know what is happening.'

She acknowledges that she can't talk about her work in social situations, because of the horror film images that are attached to the job. So she usually says, 'I work in a hospital', from which it is assumed that she *is* a nurse!

Good practice

Doing a professional job as a mortuary technician means being conscientious and always striving to make the body look the best it can, whatever the circumstances. While a level of control over one's emotions is necessary, there will always be the potential for upset, when it is important to talk to someone.

Although contact with the parents may be minimal, it is essential to stay aware of the emotional impact on the parents of having their child in the mortuary, whether 'at rest' awaiting the funeral director, or coping with a post-mortem. Helping to reduce the stress for parents means keeping the body for as short a time as possible, and preparing the parents for any physical changes in the child's appearance.

The mortuary technician quoted above, who is obviously proud of her work and finds it rewarding, summarised her approach to the job as follows:

> 'You need to have respect for life in order to work with the dead. You need to be able to empathise with others while controlling your own emotions. This job has to be done – so it should be done well.'

NURSES
Involvement
All the areas quoted above for hospital doctors will also apply to hospital nurses. The primary nurse, a named nurse on the ward with whom parents can identify, will have a very close involvement with child and family. In the case of death after chronic illness, nurses are likely to have built up intimate relationships over many years.

Neonatal nurses naturally become very attached to the babies in their care.

As a member of a primary healthcare team in the community, the nurse will be known to the family of a child who is terminally ill with cancer or a congenital abnormality.

Function
The nurse in casualty will form part of the emergency care team and, when the child dies, will have specific tasks relating to the laying out of the body. A senior nurse takes on responsibility for looking after the parents. Intensive care nurses are similarly required to carry out different roles, of technician before the death and comforter afterwards. Palliative care nurses work to ensure the control of pain and to see that the child is comfortable.

Overall, the nurse administers and monitors the care plan and has a pivotal role regarding communication between parents and consultants. Whether the child dies at home or hospital, the parents are always seen as the main carers, and the professional role is advising and supporting them. Hospital nurses tend to become experts in disease, while community nurses develop expertise in ongoing support.

Concerns

The need for staff support is a big issue. Road traffic accidents and cot deaths are particularly harrowing, especially when the child is unmarked and looks perfectly normal. The laying out should not be done alone. Being with bereaved parents in the rawness of their grief is very stressful and emotionally draining. In some hospitals now there is a trained staff counsellor as well as peer support.

Management issues such as staffing quotas and time allocation create extra pressures. A ward nurse cannot give two hours to be with newly bereaved parents unless this is a priority for management too.

Many nurses are concerned with what to say to a dying child and how to answer their questions, especially when parents seek to protect them from the truth. Close contact can draw the professional into family friction and squabbles.

Community paediatric nurses can feel quite isolated if there is no built-in support, particularly if a home death happens at a weekend when hospital support systems are limited.

Good practice

Discussions with nurses experienced in accident and emergency, intensive care and palliative care highlight the importance of training in interpersonal skills to deal with the emotional demands of working with loss and grief. General guidelines which emerge are:
➤ be yourself: this includes being prepared to show feelings
➤ be honest: answer questions simply and truthfully and be prepared to say 'I don't know' rather than invent answers
➤ listen to what parents want, and always try to see the situation from their point of view.

More practical points at the time of death include:
➤ allowing the family to stay with the dead child for as long as they want

- explaining that the child will get cold and change colour
- encouraging the parents to wash and dress the child
- if the child has to stay in hospital, reassure the parents they are welcome to return.

Parents also welcome the opportunity to visit the ward and talk to the nurses after the funeral.

Being informed about procedures following a death and the options available to parents is essential, and every ward should be equipped with a written protocol for staff and information leaflets for parents.

MIDWIVES
Involvement
The status of the midwife gives her a special kind of authority and significance for parents. She may well be the first to discover or confirm the loss of a fetal heartbeat. She will be involved with late miscarriages and the delivery of a baby who has died *in utero*, and with a stillbirth of a previously well baby who suffers birth complications.

Anticipated stillbirths tend to be the responsibility of senior midwives. In the event of an early cot death, the community midwife may still be visiting the mother before handing over to the health visitor.

Function
The midwife has a key role to play in the management of perinatal death and support of the parents. She works in partnership with the mother and consultant, which gives her an interpretive role, balancing medical needs with parental wishes. She prepares the mother for what will happen and keeps her informed of what is happening. After stillbirth, the midwife has a vital part to play in helping the parents face the reality of the death. This includes the now standard procedures of taking photographs, handprints, and encouraging the parents to touch and hold the baby. It is also a listening role, giving permission to the parents to express feelings. Midwives who recognise the importance of parents seeing their malformed baby have discovered the reassurance this provides. They will find beauty in their baby somewhere, and without this opportunity will see a monster in their minds.

Fathers have traditionally been excluded from this kind of care, and may need encouragement – perhaps from a male staff member – to take advantage of the opportunities to see and handle the dead baby. Fathers who do not wish to see the baby may need help to understand the importance of this ritual for the mother.

On a practical level, the midwife is well placed to explain all the procedures to parents regarding registration, post-mortem and funeral arrangements.

Concerns

As midwifery is about being productive, the death of a baby represents total failure. The midwife will experience her own grief, guilt and anger, which means dealing with her own feelings as well as those of the parents.

The loss of a twin presents a very difficult situation. The tendency is to encourage the parents to concentrate on their joy for the live birth, but if they do not grieve for the dead one, problems arise about rejecting the surviving twin.

In hospitals without separate rooms for grieving parents, it is a dilemma whether to care for them on a ward with babies, or on a ward with no babies. Once the mother is discharged home, the caring midwife may be left anxious about continuing support.

Good practice

Much work has been done in recent years to implement the recommendations and guidelines published by the Stillbirth and Neonatal Death Society (SANDS). These emphasise the importance of giving parents information, choices and time to make their own decisions.

Parents often do not know what is possible. Decisions in which parents should be involved include the following:

➤ whether and when the mother should be induced when the baby has died in the womb
➤ whether and when life-support is withdrawn if the baby is born alive but known to be dying
➤ whether to see, hold, wash and dress the dead baby
➤ whether to have a post-mortem
➤ whether to take the baby home
➤ how long the mother stays in hospital.

Involving fathers, and sometimes siblings or grandparents, is now the norm in most up-to-date maternity units. Millie and Derek, whose son Ben was stillborn, will always be grateful to their midwife for her patience and sensitivity:

> 'When she first asked us if we wanted to see him, we said no – we were feeling so tired and wretched. The next day she asked us again, but I was frightened what he would look like, and Derek didn't want me to get more upset. When my mum came, the midwife asked if she wanted to see the baby, which she did, and then that gave us the courage to see him. She brought him in to us, and we held him and cried together and felt like a proper family.'

In the absence of a birth or death certificate, some hospitals issue their own 'certificates' to acknowledge the baby's life. Most maternity units now have a written protocol, which gives priority to parents' wishes, and many now have a separate room or suite where both parents can sleep over to spend time privately with their baby.

An experienced midwife adds a word of caution about checklists: 'They can't tell you what to say. You have to treat everyone as an individual and be sensitive to their needs.'

PARAMEDICS

Involvement

Paramedics are often the first emergency responders on the scene, minutes after the fatal accident, onset of acute illness or discovery of the dead child. The way they carry out their duties can make a significant contribution to how the family copes subsequently.

Ambulance crews are trained in resuscitation and paramedics are qualified to administer drugs. One paramedic in London had dealt with 10 child deaths in five years; another could recall four in 18 years. The typical pattern of response is a 999 call through the radio control system, administering resuscitation or treatment at the scene as appropriate, and transporting the child to the hospital accident and emergency department, or directly to the mortuary if the death has been certified at home.

Function

The arrival of the ambulance is seen as a source of hope, and the paramedic as a saviour. When there is indeed hope of the child's life being saved, the obvious priority is emergency treatment and hospitalisation. When the child is already dead, however, it is usually the paramedic who is the first professional to confirm the fact. It is necessary for the parents to hear this unambiguous statement if they are to begin to take in the reality of what has happened. The priority is now the care and comfort of the parents and family.

In the case of sudden death at home, the ambulance crew will have a vital role to play in co-ordinating initial support. This may involve contacting the other parent, relatives, GP, clergy and explaining why the police must attend. As the first on the scene after a cot death, their reassurance to parents that the death was not preventable is invaluable.

Concerns

As paramedics are trained for action, it is hard to deal with the feelings of uselessness when the child has died at home. They are faced with extreme family reactions, which are unpredictable. Later, they have their own reactions to deal with, including 'there but for the grace of God goes one of mine'. If they seek help to come to terms with their own feelings over and above the informal support available from colleagues, they risk being seen as weak and inadequate. Perhaps the greatest fear is being called to a home death that involves suspected child abuse. This situation calls for great restraint to cope with the anger that arises when the basic instinct of saving life has been betrayed.

Good practice

The following pointers have been drawn from the experience of a county training officer in the ambulance service and a reference manual published by the Irish Sudden Infant Death Association:

> 'Sensitivity, common sense and good communication skills are valuable for the initial support of parents immediately after the death. These are shown by:
> - treating the child with respect and referring to him by name
> - offering practical help and comfort to the family
> - being generous with time and not hurrying a dead child away
> - explaining the bodily changes which may occur during or after the dying process, such as discolouration
> - explaining what will happen and where, reassuring parents that they can see and hold the child again at hospital

- always taking mother or nearest relative with the child in the ambulance and encouraging her to hold the child.

Support for paramedics affected by distress and trauma is part of building up good working practices and relationships with fellow officers and other colleagues in the health service.'

PATHOLOGISTS
Involvement
Although not directly involved with the child, the pathologist plays a crucial role in helping clinicians towards a diagnosis and appropriate treatment. The other area of involvement is the very intimate connection with the dead child in performing an examination of the body when a post-mortem is required. This in turn may lead to responding to requests from parents to discuss and explain the findings of the post-mortem, and to write post-mortem reports for the hospital clinicians and for the coroner if required. A coroner may request the pathologist to attend the court to speak about the findings to the inquest where the family is present.

Further, the pathologist may have an important connection to the future: for example, in helping to discover what went wrong with a failed pregnancy, so that parents can make informed choices about future pregnancies; and in contributing to the research which will help children in the future with life-threatening diseases.

One pathologist comments that, at every stage of his involvement, 'the whole driving force behind my work is to help the child and the family'.

Function
The scientific curiosity which may inspire this choice of profession is geared towards the benefit of others. Laboratory assistants perform the skilled tasks of preparing slides of tissue from biopsies and surgical procedures for the pathologist to study and interpret. Then, as part of a multi-disciplinary team, the pathologist will contribute these findings to help colleagues form an accurate diagnosis to report to parents and to inform treatment decisions. Sometimes a biopsy result will be needed immediately, while the child is undergoing surgery, so that the surgeons know what kind of tumour they are dealing with, for example, and what action to take.

A post-mortem of a child or baby may be requested by the parents, or it can be legally required when the death was unexpected, whether from illness, accident or violence.

The pathologist will have a mortuary technician to help in the process of following the routine procedures involved with a post-mortem examination. The pathology report that results from this examination is designed to explain the cause(s) of death and the mode of death, if possible, to clinicians, parents, and to the coroner. A written report goes to the coroner a few weeks before the inquest, and the coroner then decides whether to call the pathologist to the court to elucidate the findings and answer any queries.

Sooner or later, and it may be much later, parents may need further clarification of the post-mortem results. Nagging questions persist and may involve future choices for the family. In such cases the pathologist's time with the parents in explaining and discussing the report can be hugely reassuring.

Concerns

Pathologists are not magicians, and one of the challenges of the job is meeting the expectations of others in overestimating the extent of available information. The perception of pathology in the public eye has been greatly influenced by dramatic media portrayals. As one pathologist said:

> 'The popular picture of the pathologist is of someone standing on the bank next to a pond where different bodies are taken out for him to identify, as in most TV programmes; or he may be seen as a cold forensic scientist who can provide amazingly detailed information'.

In the professional domain, pathologists can be underestimated by colleagues who are ignorant of the skilled work they do, since pathology is not routinely covered in medical training. Having one's contribution valued is then all the more rewarding! The status of the pathology department is often reflected in the space and resources allocated within the Trust. An improvement in resources was one outcome as a result of the organ retention scandals to hit some hospitals in the late 1990s. The bad publicity that resulted from the unethical practice of a few rogue practitioners was very damaging to the profession, but this effect has thankfully receded with time, and the general attitude is now much less hostile and more understanding.

An understandable concern for anyone entering the profession is the emotional toll of conducting post-mortem examinations on babies and children. Perhaps this is where it helps that the pathologist has not had a continuing relationship with the child as a dying patient. The strong emotions expressed at an inquest can also be challenging.

Good practice
Finding one's own support strategies is therefore essential. A seasoned pathologist at a leading paediatric hospital remarked:

> 'Even after 30 years, I still feel emotionally drained after doing one or two post-mortems in a day. I need to walk out in the fresh air, or listen to a piece of Bach, to give me back my serenity.'

His top recommendations for good practice were as follows:
➤ be professional
➤ be humble and honest
➤ communicate well with colleagues
➤ keep your emotional responses under control
And, above all:
➤ never forget that the subject and object of the job is a sick child and an anxious family.

POLICE
Involvement
Child deaths involving the police are all sudden and traumatic: accidents, murders, suicides and cot deaths. They involve the police officer in unwelcome tasks, and require behaving with great tact, dignity and compassion. The inability to rescue a child from a house fire is reported to be particularly harrowing, as indeed it is for firefighters.

Function
It is the police function to report to the coroner any sudden death where the deceased has not been seen by a doctor in the previous month, or if the cause of death is uncertain. This is not generally appreciated, so the involvement of the police in the event of a cot death has to be explained carefully. The investigating officer's task is to enquire into the circumstances of the death, view the body and have the child identified prior to hospitalisation for post-mortem. The removal of bedding and clothing to help with the

pathologist's report needs to be handled with sensitivity.

'Giving the death message' is a police term for delivering news that a death has occurred, and is considered harder than dealing with the victim of an accident. The unexpected police officer knocking at the door is the stereotypical dread of all parents.

Where criminal investigations are concerned, ongoing contact with the family to keep them fully informed is not always seen as a priority for the police, but is vital to the parents.

Concerns

Delivering news of a child's death causes great anxiety about what to say and the reactions of the parents. Shifting attitudes away from the 'stiff upper lip' have brought a recognition of the distress and need to debrief afterwards with a senior or welfare officer.

Being asked for details of traumatic deaths is also stressful, with uncertainty about how much to say. There is a natural wish to protect parents, especially the mother, from unpleasant facts, and an inclination to defer to another person or later time. This can leave parents frustrated and resentful.

Seeking help for stress can be seen as a sign of weakness, with concerns about confidentiality if ongoing support is required to cope with personal reactions.

Good practice

Police forces all over the country are now recognising the importance of preparing officers for these traumatic situations, with sessions of 'breaking bad news' and 'talking to parents' being included in training programmes. The experiences of bereaved parents underline the importance of the following.

➤ Avoid protecting parents: they need to see and to know in order to grieve.

➤ Answer questions as honestly as possible.

➤ Involve both parents and keep the family together.

➤ Treat the family as you would like your own to be dealt with in similar circumstances.

➤ Wear plain clothes in sensitive situations, such as home visits after a cot death.

➤ Give parents time with their child: do not hurry them.

➤ Always refer to the child or baby by name.

Being well-informed helps. The officer feels more confident and the family reassured if they are clear about legal requirements, post-mortem and inquest procedures. The Foundation for the Study of Infant Deaths and the Scottish Cot Death Trust publish excellent information leaflets for police officers.

Every force has designated staff who take on a welfare role. Some forces have organised a system of peer counsellors from all levels of staff to encourage officers to talk about their feelings after involvement with traumatic incidents.

REGISTRARS OF BIRTHS, MARRIAGES AND DEATHS
Involvement
The registrar of a medium-sized town (population 150 000) can expect to deal with one or two deaths of children per month. Registration normally takes place in the district where the child died. The informants, usually the parents, can now register the death in *any* Register Office in England and Wales. A statutory declaration is signed and then forwarded to the office in the district where the death occurred. This service may involve a slight delay before the relevant certificate can be issued, but is obviously helpful to all concerned when the death occurs a long way from home. Some registrars go out to maternity hospitals to register stillbirths and neonatal deaths, and this facility is much appreciated by shocked and grieving parents.

Function
The role of the registrar is to perform the legal requirement of recording information about the death, including data for statistics, and administering the paperwork relating to the disposal of the body. In this sense the registrar is accountable to the relevant government department – the general register office. The legislation concerning who can register, and where the registration takes place, does not allow for a mobile population.

Concerns
The main concern is getting the registration done while parents are in distress. Spelling out the details of the child's death and seeing them recorded in black and white for the first time can be a gruelling experience for parents, and the registrar has to guide them through the form-filling in an emotionally charged atmosphere.

Surprisingly, there is at present no statutory training for registrars in dealing with bereaved relatives. However there is a growing acceptance among registrars of the idea of a bereavement pathway and that they play a significant part in this process.

Good practice

As defined by a parent:

> 'We went together to register Barry's death. There were several people waiting but the receptionist showed us to a small private room till the registrar was ready to see us. He was very courteous – said he was sorry about the reason for coming, and explained what had to be done. When Susan got upset, he put his pen down and waited till we were ready to go on. He checked he'd got all the details right, then gave us two copies of the death certificate. It may seem a little thing, but it was pleasing to see such nice handwriting.'

A registrar's comments:

> 'It's important to explain clearly to parents what my task is, and then I try to ask the questions as sensitively as possible. For example, I have to ask whether the informant was present at the death. The bureaucratic version is: "Were you present at the death?" But I prefer to ask: "Were you able to be present at the death?", which takes into account their experience in a more human way. I make a point of using the baby's or child's name as often as possible, as a mark of respect.'

SOCIAL WORKERS

Involvement

Fieldworkers will meet child death only rarely, when the affected family is already being supported or where a child is subject to child protection procedures.

The hospital social worker will be closely involved as part of the care team in both acute and ongoing situations, and may be the one person who remains constant to the family throughout the treatment process.

Function

The hospital social worker's primary role is to support the family and to be an advocate for the parents. This support is available to all families, regardless of status, and facilitates communication between patient, parents and staff. Advocacy means representing the parents' wishes and concerns, and acting as an interpreter and mediator; it requires good counselling skills. The counselling function can continue well into the first year of bereavement and beyond, with home visits and facilitating group support.

Practical support includes providing information about benefits and entitlements during terminal illness, helping with transport and family care at the time of the death and guiding the parents through the first days of bereavement. As well as providing information about legalities, the social worker is ideally placed to help the parents make informed choices about the funeral and to consider the needs of other family members. There may be some overlap here with the midwife, health visitor or community nurse, depending on existing relationships, making good communication essential and maybe indicating a co-ordinating role with other professionals and agencies.

Concerns

Those who have opted to work in areas with a high incidence of mortality, such as casualty or intensive care, are vulnerable to accumulated stress and need well-developed support and supervision systems. Operating as a buffer between families and professionals can also be very taxing.

Child protection social workers are faced with acute dilemmas and anxieties when the life of a child is thought to be at risk. When a child dies as a result of neglect or abuse, the professional is left with feelings of anger, helplessness and guilt, and needs intense support. Such support may be difficult to access in a situation where external and internal investigations dictate the removal of files, the suspension of workers directly involved, and an injunction not to discuss the case. High-profile cases invite vilification by the press, particularly when the child was on the 'at risk' register and subject to the monitoring of social care professionals.

Good practice

Social workers in the hospital setting have to be willing to undertake bereavement work, be aware of the effects of grief for themselves and others, and be prepared to work in a multidisciplinary way. A commitment to the rights of parents and the advocacy role underpin all good practice. One maternity unit social worker comments:

> 'I aim to work towards parents feeling that everything that could be done, was done, and that they may be left with as few regrets as possible. If they can say this, it makes their grieving easier.'

Counselling skills are basic to all social work, although the level of sensitivity needed for this emotive area indicates the benefits of further training. In order to use these skills effectively, there needs to be an acceptance within their management structure that bereavement support is part of good working practice.

Above all, the social worker is valued by parents as a good listener and as someone who can reduce their isolation. When Jo's baby David died, the GP gave them the telephone number of the hospital social worker:

> 'This was my first glimmer of hope . . . and I clutched that phone number for two weeks before making contact. She just let us talk. She introduced us to a support group of bereaved parents. They too carried a big ball of black pain around – what a relief it was to meet them.'

TEACHERS (*see also* Chapters 6 and 8)
Involvement
The whole school community is deeply affected when a pupil dies, and teachers are indirectly involved when a pupil's sibling or young friend dies. The staff of specialist schools for children with life-threatening conditions include physiotherapists, occupational therapists and domestic personnel as well as teachers. Hospital teachers form significant relationships with children who are terminally ill.

Function
The class teacher forms an important link between school and family when a child is hospitalised, keeping the child in touch with peers and the normality of school life. When the child dies, teachers provide models for pupils in how they react. A senior teacher may well take the lead in liaising with parents, formally acknowledging the death in school, and facilitating some

ceremony or ritual to express the school's mourning. Practical tasks include amending class lists and collecting anything belonging to the child.

In the case of sudden death, teachers will have more extreme reactions to deal with as shockwaves run through the school, causing anger and anxiety.

Bereaved siblings present teachers with another challenge of what to say and how to accommodate their grief. Trusted teachers may be required to act as a counsellor and confidante for the child, or even for the parents. In the rare cases when more is required, the teacher is ideally placed to monitor the reactions of the grieving child, alert the parents and enlist specialist help.

Concerns

The effects of a teenage suicide are particularly traumatic and teachers may be concerned about aroused curiosity and copycat attempts. In fact, any cloak of silence increases the students' anxiety. Fears of hysterical reactions may also smother open acknowledgement of any sudden death. (For guidance on suicide and young people, *see* Chapter 8, pp 177–9, *Support for schools*.)

A death that occurs during holidays presents special problems as to how to handle the news on return to school. If a death occurs on a school trip or organised educational holiday, when teachers are *in loco parentis*, extensive debriefing and counselling will be required.

Teachers are not always informed that a pupil has lost a sibling, which makes it difficult to respond appropriately to any problematic reactions.

Good practice

Any school that exposes students to death as a natural part of life, through nature studies, biology, personal and social education programmes, will be better placed to deal openly with the unnatural death of a child. Many secondary schools now include 'death studies' on the pastoral curriculum, and devote some in-service training time to preparing teachers by looking at their own attitudes to death. Younger children may need help with the difference between death and sleep, and are able to cope better with clear, unambiguous answers to questions (*see* Chapter 6). Many good books for all ages are now on the market to help children make sense of their experience (*see* Appendix C).

In practical terms, the eventuality of child death should be included in the school protocol, with clear guidelines as to who does what. Acknowledging the death is always important. Teachers should keep any of the child's work for parents to collect, if they so wish.

Head teachers, or those with special responsibility for pastoral care, need to consider ways and means of communicating information about a dying child, or the death of a child, which will impact on their pupils. While confidentiality has to be respected, good liaison with parents and the school health service or community paediatrician will make it easier to confront such a sensitive situation.

A primary school teacher offers the benefit of her experience in the loss of a pupil who died from leukaemia:

> 'When he returned to school after his transplant, I tried to treat him as normally as possible. At the same time, I kept in close contact with the parents, and the children helped to organise a sponsored swim for leukaemia research. They wrote to him and visited during his last illness. When he died, the children were told in a calm and honest way. Many of us cried and I felt it important that I did not hide my grief.'

A senior secondary teacher offers this advice to colleagues:

> 'Never underestimate pupils' feelings, as siblings or friends, and don't underestimate your own influence for good. Listen to them, and try to understand beyond the words: they may ask for your help in a roundabout way. It takes courage.'

References

Department of Health. *When a Patient Dies: advice on developing bereavement services in the NHS.* London: HM Government; 2005. Available at: www.dh.gov.uk/en/Publicationsandstatistics/Publications/PublicationsPolicyAndGuidance/DH_4122191 (accessed 26 June 2009).

Lendrum S, Syme G. *Gift of Tears.* London: Routledge; 1992.

CHAPTER 4

Guidelines for all

'Give sorrow words; the grief that does not speak
Whispers the o'er-fraught heart, and bids it break.'
Malcolm to Macduff when he had received news
of his wife and children's murders.

Macbeth Act IV, Scene III

We do not have to be experts to support people with their grief. What we can all do to help is to assess their needs and our abilities to provide what they need.

This includes being able to explain what we can offer as well as what we can't. It involves being a reflective practitioner in whatever we do. It means knowing the limits of our own competence and knowing where and when to refer people on to other services.

Having said that, there are general principles that apply to all, and that supply the helper with more confidence. Sensitivity and compassion are developed rather than taught, but there are skills that can be practised. The importance of support for the helper cannot be overstated, and the purpose of supervision will be discussed. Training needs are covered by the suggested contents of a training programme, including awareness-raising, listening skills and some helping strategies. Finally, all readers are invited to address themselves to the resources questionnaire at the end of the chapter.

GENERAL PRINCIPLES

Regardless of role or situation, the most basic principle is the importance of *listening to what individual people say they want rather than presuming what they need*. After that, it is useful to bear in mind the themes that run through the experience of families quoted in this book. Families say they want: information, choices, control and permission to grieve.

Being there is more important than what you do; listening is more important than talking

There is often pressure to know the right things to say, and a fear of saying the wrong things. We can end up feeling so anxious that we cannot listen! Be assured that simply by being in attendance or by making your visit you are doing something useful. If you are offering emotional support by listening as well, then you are doing a great deal. You are conveying the messages that the family is *not* carrying a social disease and that you are not afraid of their pain.

You are still going to feel pretty helpless, but it is important to recognise that as a feature of bereavement support, and not to let the feeling of helplessness prevent your making contact. More about attending and listening skills can be found on pages 102–3.

Be clear about your involvement

You need to be clear about your role and what support you are offering. This should then be made clear to the bereaved person, even if your professional title appears to make it obvious. Are you there as part of your job, or out of personal concern? Are you representing an agency? Is this a one-off contact or are you offering ongoing care? Are you offering practical or emotional support? At the outset, a named introduction is a common courtesy, and it is good practice to leave behind some written confirmation of who you are and where you can be contacted.

These may well be routine procedures, but they take on added importance in bereavement when people commonly feel impotent and confused. The newly bereaved may be particularly vulnerable to people who are keen to peddle their own belief systems. Remember, too, that many bereaved parents lose faith in any justice in the world and are sensitive to further disappointment. The helper therefore needs to be scrupulous about keeping appointments, keeping time and promising only what is realistic in terms of further support.

The issue of confidentiality also needs to be considered carefully.

Reassurance should be given that private information will be treated sensitively, and that any information shared is strictly in the interests of the bereaved person. Sort out with your supervisor the conditions, if any, that would compromise confidentiality.

Use the child's name

This means so much to parents, for the name keeps alive the memory of this child. It is an acknowledgement that the child really existed at a time when it is difficult for parents to separate reality from fantasy. Saying the name also means that you are interested in the child, whether or not you knew him, and that you recognise the meaning of the child's absence. It can be tempting to tiptoe round the child, in the mistaken belief that mentioning him will upset the parent. A moment's reflection is sufficient to realise that the grief for the child is ever-present, that being 'upset' is entirely appropriate and that this response arises from our own fear of painful feelings getting in the way. Asking about the child, looking at photographs and mementoes are ways of paying respect to child and parent, and help to facilitate expression of grief.

Avoid platitudes and euphemisms

Having respect for another person, regardless of age, race and social background, is one of the core conditions for a helping relationship. Respect can be shown for the other person's feelings, thoughts and beliefs, whether or not one agrees with them. Lack of respect is shown in patronising comments, discounting remarks, moralising and platitudes.

A platitude is defined as 'an empty remark made as if it were important'. To apply well-worn phrases that so easily miss the mark is insulting. Using any phrase that begins with 'At least . . .' only serves to undermine the bereaved person's suffering. Sadly, parents hear them all too often: 'At least you have two other healthy children' or 'At least you are young enough to have another child.'

A euphemism is a device for describing something unpleasant in milder terms in an attempt to avoid the unpleasantness. Death is riddled with euphemisms such as 'We've lost him' and 'He passed away'. It has already been pointed out how mischievous such phrases can be for children, and that their persistent use may indicate continuing denial of the reality of the death. Euphemisms should not be used by carers and helpers because they can cause misunderstanding and because they avoid reality. There is no way of dressing up the harsh fact of death.

Each bereavement is unique

First, it helps to remember that each child is a unique individual. Even a premature baby will have unique characteristics. All the particular features of the child need to be mourned, and as the child is often idealised by the parents, which is not to deny the special courage of many terminally ill children, you may be able to help them grieve for the whole child, warts and all.

Second, it is important to recognise each bereaved person as an individual and to allow them the uniqueness of their own loss without constant comparisons with others' experiences or, worse still, your own. This denies the bereaved person the opportunity to be seen and accepted for herself. Out of this attention to the individual comes the ability to see more clearly the world through her eyes. Empathy is another of the core conditions that encourage trust in a helping relationship.

People come before theory. An understanding of patterns and common features is valuable: it serves to reassure you, and shared experience is comforting for the bereaved. But you can never presume to know how it is, so avoid saying, 'I know how you feel'.

It is also useful to remember that everything has to be done again by the parents and family for the first time after the child's death – the first meal, the first visit to a supermarket, the first Christmas, the first holiday.

Seeing is believing

It is difficult to accept the reality of death, and more so if a healthy child dies suddenly. Those who grieve a personal loss need to see some evidence to connect what they understand in their heads with what they know in their hearts. Parents want to say goodbye and feel physically close in death. Parents have the right to see their dead child, however shocking or distressing that may be. They need preparation more than protection. Your patient understanding may be required in helping them consider the pros and cons, with time to make an informed choice (*see* Chapter 1, pp 10–11; Chapter 3, p 81; Chapter 5, pp 114–16).

The same general principle applies to whether siblings should be encouraged or discouraged to see the dead child. Children are often resentful later if they were not given the choice. Very often, children are protected from knowing the full extent of the last illness and from seeing the dying child in the last hours. Even children of a very young age benefit from being included in the reality of the situation. These sensitive issues are for the parents to resolve, but they may ask for your help in thinking them through.

Fantasy is worse than reality

Knowledge is power, and having information gives one a greater sense of control in any situation. When parental responsibility is involved, the need for information is paramount. The paternalism of the medical profession is thankfully giving way to an understanding of how important it is to keep parents fully involved and consulted.

As well as being ethically correct, this enables parents to work through their reactions to the death. What is not known will be imagined, and almost invariably the fantasy turns out to be worse than the reality. Younger children have the doubtful advantage of literal imagination, which can be very confusing and worrying for them if they hear only half a story and if questions are not answered honestly (*see* Chapter 6, pp 124–6).

Involve all the family

At the time of the death the mother is often protected from harsh realities, but afterwards she tends to be the focus of attention. Ask directly after the welfare of the father and other children too. If your advice and help are sought in the practical arrangements for the funeral and other rituals, remember the benefits if all the family can be involved. Parents, children and grandparents are much more likely to be able to support each other in their grief later if they have felt included in decisions about the form of service, the wording on a wreath or headstone, and what happens to the child's possessions.

There are no experts

Of course there are those who have more experience of dealing with child death and bereaved families, and those whose training equips them for special tasks. But in most situations the person best qualified to offer support is someone who is already known and trusted by the family. Bereavement work makes everyone feel inadequate and it is tempting to look around for an 'expert' who can do a better job. The only experts on this unique experience are the family. Being supportive is much more about being there, rather than doing something. You will, however, need support and supervision for a variety of reasons.

You will need support

If you were involved with the child's care before the death or at the time of death, you will need some outlet for your own reactions. Feelings of failure and helplessness need to be expressed without fear of being judged as inadequate. Sensitive support of bereaved families is stressful and requires recognition of the demands being made of you. You may find yourself affected on several levels: by the family's grief, by memories of your own losses, by fears for the future, by anger and frustration at feeling so powerless to help. *If these feelings are not safely discharged, you either risk your own mental health or compromise your capacity for compassion.* You may be lucky enough to have instant support available among colleagues, but if you are working in isolation it is essential to have time built into your work schedule to offload. This may be combined with supervision from someone responsible for overseeing your work (*see* below).

The learning points from these general principles are now summarised and offered as a check against your own experience:
➤ show your concern by being there for the family
➤ listen more than you talk
➤ be clear about what you are offering
➤ be courteous and considerate
➤ use the child's name
➤ encourage the family to talk about the child
➤ avoid meaningless platitudes
➤ respect the uniqueness of the family's experience
➤ enable the family to make informed choices
➤ pay attention to brothers and sisters
➤ encourage the family to share decisions
➤ do not underestimate the value of your support
➤ get support for yourself.

SUPERVISION

Supervision means different things to different people. It can be used for monitoring, assessment, evaluation and support. Many professionals have supervision of their practice as a matter of course, often with their line manager. In counselling and psychotherapy, supervision is an essential requirement to practice, with established guidelines that seek to separate supervision from line management.

The primary purpose of supervision in relation to therapeutic work with an individual or with a group concerns the well-being of the client or group members. Supervision aims to address the question: how can the needs of the client or service user be best met? At one step removed from the actual work, the supervisor aims to support the worker in achieving this end.

Why is supervision of bereavement work so important?

➤ Being so close to death is stressful. When the death is that of a child, and when the death is sudden, the added dimensions of tragedy and trauma make this a very difficult area of work.
➤ Working with death and bereavement tends to be isolating, reflecting the lonely experience of grief itself.
➤ Supporting someone in grief can cause a blurring of personal and professional boundaries.
➤ Child death may involve litigation issues.

What are the functions of supervision?

The functions of supervision generally fall into three categories.
1 *Supportive*: to provide moral, psychological and emotional support for the worker.
2 *Educative*: to facilitate learning and understanding, to develop skills and resources.
3 *Managerial*: (with a small 'm') to clarify roles, tasks and boundaries.

All three functions have clear application to bereavement support work: whether as counsellor, befriender, church visitor, health visitor, family worker; and whether working with individuals, couples, families or groups.

The *supportive* aspects are paramount. The supervisor provides a safety net for workers to identify and discharge their own feelings and reactions. These may be in relation to their personal experience of loss and bereavement; their experience of children or their own childhood; their achievements and frustrations in this area of work. Feelings of sadness, helplessness and inadequacy, which are appropriate to this work, can be safely explored to prevent a protective blunting of emotions at one extreme and over-identification with the bereaved person's reactions at the other extreme. The supervisor helps the worker to monitor her own well-being. Supervision provides the space where the demands of the work can be appreciated and the efforts of the worker are valued.

The *educative* aspects integrate theory with practice, by looking together at the skills and interventions used, and by considering the relationships that underpin the work. The role of the supervisor here is to help the worker identify learning and develop further insights; to guide and inform about alternative strategies and resources; and to make sense of unfolding processes. Thus the supervisee learns to work within her level of competence and to develop her competence. The ongoing evaluation of skills, experience and training needs benefits the worker as well as the client.

The *managerial* aspects relate more to the self-management of the worker than to institutional management, though agency issues are bound to impact on the work. Managerial supervision tasks include the assessment of needs and resources; the clarification of roles; the setting of objectives; time boundaries; and ethical issues such as confidentiality and client safety. Liaison with other people and referral to other agencies may need to be considered. The supervisor's role in the managerial sense is usually to monitor, advise and co-ordinate. However, on rare occasions of questionable ethics or malpractice on the part of the worker, the supervisor is responsible for giving clear direction or for taking further action to deal with the situation.

Where can you get supervision?

If bereavement support forms a significant part of your work, you should have regular, individual supervision sessions with someone who has substantial experience in this field and is familiar with the issues. Preferably that person should be someone who is not also your line manager. If it has to be your line manager, then you should have a separate agreement for meeting together for supervision purposes, which sets this work apart from other line management functions. The major argument for supervision to be provided by someone external to the agency or employment structure is that workers should be free to explore personal issues and to own feelings of inadequacy.

Whoever provides the supervision, obvious qualifications include experience of a supervisory role and training in supervision; a working knowledge of loss and bereavement issues; and an understanding of child development and family dynamics. When the supervision involves groups, a working knowledge of group dynamics needs to be added to the list.

Some of the supervisory functions listed above can be performed in a supervision group. Such a group can be made up of colleagues within the same work setting, or it can have a multidisciplinary membership of professionals or volunteers concerned with similar issues. A group of experienced people can run this as a peer group very successfully, though without an objective facilitator some of the benefits and requirements of supervision are lost. Where resources permit, the ideal situation includes both peer group supervision and individual supervision.

TRAINING

There is a strong case to be argued for loss and bereavement issues to be included in any basic training course in the health and caring professions, so that everyone has an opportunity to prepare mentally. Specialist short courses follow more naturally when some experience has been acquired.

The starting point for any training input is raising awareness of the personal anxieties that threaten to get in the way of dealing compassionately with others. The taboos associated with death in the Western world can be challenged only by confronting our fears and prejudices.

Awareness

Reflecting on our own losses enables us to:

➤ identify reactions and ways of coping, which give insights into others' experiences
➤ recognise areas of loss that have been difficult to resolve
➤ realise that working with someone grieving a similar loss will trigger associated reactions to our past and feared losses
➤ acknowledge the difficulty of dealing with death in terms of our own mortality.

Acknowledging concerns that commonly beset those who support the bereaved is a reassuring exercise. Such concerns include:

➤ how will I cope?
➤ will I get sucked into others' distress?
➤ I won't know what to say or do
➤ should I show my feelings?

Acknowledgement of our own limitations helps to make these anxieties more manageable. A sense of vocation is associated with professions that seek to heal, empower, develop and support other people. It is therefore important to be prepared for the following feelings:

➤ feeling powerless to help
➤ a sense of failure and even guilt
➤ being inadequate for the task.

These reactions belong to the nature of grief. They do not deny the value of your support and care.

SKILLS

The two foundation skills required for bereavement support are basic to all effective communication: attending and listening. They are, of course, interrelated. Both sound simple but can be extremely difficult in practice, particularly when dealing with painful feelings. The learning points summarised below are best made by setting up exercises that allow participants to experience the effects of good and bad practice.

Attending

Paying attention means being alert to someone and being interested in what they have to say, which communicates the message that they are of value. That in itself encourages trust and free expression, and has a healing effect. Attending means suspending one's own concerns and prejudices, and being in a state of 'not knowing'. As well as conveying respect, attending also enables the listener to observe the whole person as communicated by body language and nonverbal behaviour. Good attention is demonstrated by:
➤ setting the scene: even before the communication starts, the way in which a person is greeted conveys respect
➤ making eye contact, which is crucial; facial expressions, nods and grunts also provide physical evidence of being attended to
➤ removing barriers such as desks, equipment and papers, and sitting at the same level
➤ avoiding distracters such as bleeps and telephones.

Listening

Listening is a complex activity. It includes:
➤ giving attention
➤ receiving information
➤ taking in the thoughts and feelings conveyed
➤ interpreting behaviour

➤ noticing key points and themes
➤ checking that you have heard and understood correctly.

The focus remains on the speaker when the listener reflects back what has been heard. Restatements, paraphrasing and summarising the messages received form an important part of the process for several reasons:
➤ the speaker is assured of your understanding
➤ if you have got it wrong, the speaker can correct you
➤ the speaker can hear the effect of what she is saying.

Listening involves considerable self-discipline. It means suspending your own assumptions, judgements, advice and solutions. It may also mean tolerating silence, allowing the speaker time and space to gather thoughts and give expression to feelings.

HELPING STRATEGIES

While active listening forms the cornerstone of bereavement support, to facilitate the expression of the disordered thoughts and feelings of grief, other approaches may be required for ongoing support. More directive strategies may also be indicated when the bereaved person finds it difficult to talk, or when uncompleted mourning tasks have been identified.

Most of the ideas that follow are simple but can be powerfully effective. A training event is the ideal opportunity to try them out on yourself and colleagues.

Prompts

Some people welcome invitations to talk about their loved one, particularly if they have been discouraged from doing so by others.

Open questions about the child might be:
➤ 'Can you tell me more about . . .?'
➤ 'What sort of child was he?'
➤ 'What are your special memories?'

Photographs and mementoes provide a fund of recollections, and a genuine interest in sharing them encourages warmth and trust.

Linking

One of the tasks of mourning is making sense of what has happened, and finding a place for the loss which offers some meaning. The bereaved may need some help in linking the past to the present, and this can be done by talking them through the process of change, perhaps in three stages.

1 Invite reminiscences of what life was like before the child died – a typical weekday, holiday and so on – for self and family.
2 Ask for a (repeat) rehearsal of the events at the time of the child's death.
3 Invite reflections on how life has changed after the child died, and how things are different now.

Rituals

Bereavement is made up of many little goodbyes, and it may be appropriate to construct together some private rituals to help the bereaved deal with difficult memories. For instance, a parent requested help with revisiting the road junction where her daughter had been killed years previously. Another parent helped her child grieve for a friend, whose funeral they had been unable to attend, by releasing helium balloons with goodbye messages on them.

Writing

For many parents and siblings, writing becomes an important therapeutic tool. When such writing can be shared, it is a powerful communicator of inner feelings.

For those who are anguished by things left unsaid to the child, the device of writing a letter, addressed as it were to the child, can be liberating. Alternatively an audio tape could be made, with messages interspersed with favourite music. Websites for posting messages provide a natural medium for a growing number of people.

Drawing

Children are less inhibited about drawing than adults, and may derive greater benefit from pictures than words. Images and colours help to give shape to memories and complex emotions.

Scrapbooks

This is another useful approach with children, but is equally valuable to adults, and a great activity in which to include all the family, or the child's school friends. Photographs, keepsakes, written memories, pictures of favourite pop stars and activities can all contribute to a shared album of memories. This may be a useful suggestion when one of the family is left with an impossibly idealised picture of the child, as the scrapbook can easily accommodate different images – the comic and the naughty as well as the sad and the good.

Memory boxes

Following on from the scrapbook idea, the advantage of a memory box is that it will accommodate three-dimensional objects. Favourite toys, video cassettes and other memorabilia associated with the child can be kept in this special place along with photographs and the written word. For some families this can be a particular comfort when the time is right to clear the child's room of his or her special effects.

Geneogram

This is a diagrammatic way of depicting the family, like a family tree, which records births, marriages and deaths and provides a tool for exploring family relationships. It is drawn up with the help of the bereaved, and is useful for gaining a wider perspective on the significance of the child's death for different family members. (*See also* Chapter 7, p 151 and Appendix D.)

RESOURCES QUESTIONNAIRE

All readers are invited to assess their resources and needs by considering these questions.

1 How does my personal experience affect my attitude to bereavement?
2 What is the level of awareness of my own actual and feared losses?
3 Can I identify the other person's needs, and the tasks involved in my support?
4 What is my role?
5 What relevant skills do I have?
6 How do I recognise my limitations? Am I being honest, or modest?
7 Do I have training needs?
8 Do I know when, how and where to refer on for more specialist help?
9 Are my needs for consultation and support being met?

Further reading

Hawkins P, Shohet R. *Supervision in the Helping Professions.* 3rd ed. Oxford: OUP; 2007.

CHAPTER 5

Guidelines for stressful situations

'I am not mad; I would to heaven I were!
For then, 'tis like I should forget myself
O, if I could, what grief should I forget!'
Constance, on the death of her son Arthur

King John Act III Scene IV

There are certain key situations when the words, actions and attitudes of professionals can have a lasting impact on the family, for good or ill. Advice may be sought by parents who are emotionally vulnerable. Others may be temporarily hostile towards those who seek to help them. Years later, parents tend to remember with utmost clarity the detail of turning points in their child's illness and treatment. And in the heightened sensitivity of their grief, thoughtless comments add to their pain just as caring gestures are treasured.

Knowing this adds to the sense of heavy responsibility at such times for professionals to 'get it right' or at least avoid 'putting one's foot in it'. Anxiety is a natural response when faced with painful emotions and a sense of helplessness. There are no blueprints for any given situation, but some general guidelines can provide signposts.

It needs to be stressed that each situation is unique and people's reactions are unpredictable. No-one can get it right all the time, but the sincerity of trying to do one's best is what matters.

BREAKING BAD NEWS

One father recalls how much it meant to him that when his son died the doctor was visibly upset at the bedside. By contrast, one mother is still outraged, 10 years later, that the doctor yawned after telling her that her daughter had just died. Another mother remembers:

> 'We held her until the Sister said "she's gone now", and I hated her so much I could have done murder – but I know I needed to hear the words to believe it.'

The task of communicating bad news is unenviable, whether at the time of diagnosis, treatment results, accident, post-mortem results or inquest. It gives rise to similar reactions as experienced when being on the receiving end: anxiety, fear, panic, anger, helplessness, failure, sadness, despair. Some of the anxiety may be about the other person's reactions, because the bearers of bad news have been known to be lynched! The message-carrier is certainly an easy target for first reactions of angry disbelief, particularly as a member of the medical profession.

A simple checklist is offered below to help identify the ideal circumstances for breaking bad news.

Why?

This may seem obvious, but the underlying question is an ethical one and raises issues of information and control. Is the amount of information given on a 'need-to-know' or 'right-to-know' basis? Nothing enrages parents more than discovering later that information about their own child has been withheld.

When?

The answer to the above will determine the timing. On a 'right-to-know' basis, the guideline must be: as soon as possible.

By whom?

Qualities are favoured more than position: ideally, it should be someone known and trusted, who shows sensitivity and has good communication skills. Most parents say it helps if the person has a continuing involvement with them, rather than someone who appears and then disappears. The importance of the authority of the person seems to depend on the nature of the information. A complex diagnosis, for example, requires specialist knowledge to answer parents' questions. In other hospital situations, the nursing staff offer more continuity.

Where?

Parents invariably recall the setting, and there is a strong association with the room and the importance of the occasion. The place should be somewhere comfortable, private and without interruption.

How?

If at all possible, the breaking of bad news should be in a face-to-face situation, and it is important to look the person in the eye. Take a few minutes before going into the situation to check your demeanour and gather your thoughts. If a mobile phone or page call is unavoidable, due consideration needs to be given to the likely impact of shock and distress.

Every effort should be made to tell both parents together. If this is not possible, another family member or friend should be present for support.

The message should be unambiguous to avoid misunderstanding, and questions should be answered as honestly as possible. Euphemisms are not helpful. In the case of giving a diagnosis of terminal illness, a balance needs to be struck between realism and hope.

Shock and disbelief may require time for the information to be received, so it is important to go at their pace. This means checking out their understanding of what you have said, and repeating or restating the information as necessary.

Check their responses: ask how they are feeling, what are their immediate concerns, are there any questions they want to ask. Some people react to bad news with denial, apparent apathy or by trivialising it, and these defences need to be respected. Before leaving the interview, ongoing support and follow-up needs to be ensured. This may involve transport arrangements, medical attention, alerting local resources and providing reassurance that there will be opportunities for addressing questions and concerns at a future time.

Finally, you will need the support of a colleague, ideally to accompany you or at least to debrief you afterwards.

Some experiences of parents

'Christine had various tests at the hospital, but we weren't told what they were for. Then one day we had a letter informing us that Christine had been diagnosed as a cystic fibrosis child and we were to visit the clinic in three weeks' time. We had no idea what cystic fibrosis was. A friend gave us the address of the Cystic Fibrosis Fund and we sent off for some leaflets.'

'We pinned all our hopes on Jason having this operation to remove the tumour. He seemed to recover very well, but the consultant was doubtful. Then Jason went downhill fast, and in the end the consultant sat down with us and said there was nothing more they could do for him. We'd got to know him quite well and it was like we were all in this together. He answered all our questions and we looked at the options. He taped that session and gave us the tape to take home: it was a great help to go over it again and play it to our parents. You can't remember half of what's said otherwise.'

'Tracy lived for 11 days. I'm usually squeamish about illness and medical things, but I wanted to know every detail about her condition. The doctor went through the post-mortem and answered all my questions as best she could – she was honest about not knowing all the answers – but it was so important for me to know all there was to know. My mum came with me, which was a help.'

'The police officer who called said that the paramedics had taken Simon to hospital and there was still hope of reviving him. It wasn't till we got to the hospital two hours later that we discovered he was dead when they found him. We felt so resentful about that lie. Did the policeman think he was doing us a favour? Our son was dead for over two hours and other people knew it and we didn't. The hospital doctor who confirmed the death was cold and detached. We wished he had shown some feeling, at least said he was sorry.'

EMERGENCY PROCEDURES AND INTENSIVE CARE

'We recognise that relatives have a part to play in our work, and that we help to create memories that will affect them for the rest of their lives.' So says the clinical nurse specialist at the accident and emergency department of Wythenshawe Hospital, Manchester, where the consultant and casualty team introduced an enlightened policy that allows parents to be involved and fully informed throughout treatment. Lack of information and involvement are the most consistent regrets and resentments of parents of children receiving emergency medical care.

Traditionally, the care of patients' relatives has been seen as a nursing issue, as death is not a medical problem. However, more and more consultants have a growing understanding of bereavement support as part of the total healthcare package. At Alder Hey Children's Hospital in Liverpool, the prevailing philosophy is that the family is the patient, not just the child. Given this commitment, traditional objections to involving the family can be faced and overcome. More hospitals in the UK now operate open access to parents, which means they need never be separated from their child.

Protocol

The unpredictability of an emergency makes it impossible to lay down any set protocol for dealing with relatives, whose reactions are not consistent. The family's trauma is matched by the frantic efforts of the staff to save the child's life. Some parents merely wish to be reassured that something is being done, while others want to be present to see exactly what is going on. However, some general principles will guide good practice for the benefit of parents and help staff deal better with the feelings of failure when a child dies.

Teamwork

The staff team, from cleaner to consultant, will need to work through their own feelings and reactions in order to adopt a team approach.

The team may also include the spiritual advisor and social worker. Good team relationships are essential to the kind of flexibility and communication required.

Identified person

Someone on the team needs to be allocated to the care of the parents, to explain what is happening and to facilitate their needs short of obstructing treatment. Parents need to be prepared and cautioned about what they will see. When parents do not wish to be present during treatment, they will need to be kept closely informed. The identified person may be allocated by role: it may be the social worker or spiritual advisor who routinely acts as parental support. A medically trained person may be thought more appropriate for answering questions and explaining treatment procedures.

Resuscitation

The attendance of parents during resuscitation is a contentious issue, and professional misgivings have to be challenged as well as respected. Common objections are:

➤ staff feel inhibited
➤ parents need protecting from seeing aggressive treatment
➤ parents get in the way
➤ staff are vulnerable to criticism.

These fears stem from being faced with other people's acute emotions and the defences erected to cope with one's own feelings.

These *can* be confronted successfully once the right of parents to attend, if they wish, is accepted. In practice, staff find that parents who attend resuscitation are more concerned with the child than the treatment.

An implication is whether parents can then be involved in the decision about when resuscitation efforts should cease, always a difficult time for staff. If, when all hope has long gone, parents are unable to face the reality, the consultant has to take professional responsibility for the decision.

There are some situations where the decision to withdraw life support is fraught with difficulty. After accident-related trauma, certain criteria to establish brain stem death have to be met, which may entail necessary delay before the life support machine can be switched off. This demands particular sensitivity in explaining the situation to parents.

For most parents, being there at the moment of death and being able to touch or hold the child are essential to feeling they did all they could, that the child was not alone among strangers, and that they were able to let him go. All family members should have an opportunity to say these goodbyes, including young siblings, as long as this is acceptable to the parents.

Practicalities

It is necessary to have a separate room for relatives, of course, but also important to have a private space where the parents can be with their child immediately after the death for as long as they wish. Their primary support person needs to be available to them during that time without pressure from colleagues to be elsewhere. Procedures and options need to be explained, with a written booklet for reference on leaving. Parents who find it difficult to leave the child may find comfort in leaving something personal with the body. It is much appreciated when staff handle and address the child with the same warmth and respect as before death.

AFTER THE DEATH

This is a time when professionals who are correctly informed and aware of the issues can be very helpful to bereaved families. Parents who are plunged into grief will usually need the guidance of the nurse, doctor, social worker or chaplain, particularly when the death was unexpected. Even families who can draw on the experience of other bereavements are unlikely to feel confi-dent of their rights and obligations when a child dies. Their need for advice and guidance is never greater than at this time, not to take control away from them but so they can make their own informed choices. The assumption should not be made, as it often is, that bereaved parents – especially the mother – are not in a fit state to make decisions.

Sudden death presents the biggest challenge. There has been no prepara-tion and there is no continuity of care. The availability of hospital social workers and chaplains will be variable. Many hospital doctors see their role finishing with the death of the child, leaving follow-up care to nursing staff or to other professionals.

Clearly the scandalous practice of organs being removed at post-mortem and retained as hospital property, without parental consent, as uncovered in 1999 at Alder Hey and other hospitals, was a betrayal of trust and a denial of human rights. Parents have been doubly bereaved and traumatised. (*See* Barbara's story, Chapter 10.)

Roles and responsibilities need to be clear

The first and most important guideline, therefore, is to ensure that adequate systems are in place, and that staff induction programmes make them known. Co-ordinated care avoids the 'rugby pass' type of management.

A designated person should be responsible for the ongoing care of parents or for co-ordinating that initial support, in line with Department of Health guidelines.

The family's GP should be informed as soon as possible as the most obvious primary care co-ordinator in the community.

Giving advice and information

Information given to parents must be accurate and consistent, with an opportunity to talk it through rather than simply being offered it in written form.

Hospital staff should be aware of cultural and religious differences, with access to translators in case of language difficulties, and to signers for the deaf.

When decisions need to be made, parents should not be hurried to suit hospital routines, and time should always be allowed for parents to change their minds.

It helps to remember that the child continues to belong to the parents, except for the coroner's brief legal 'ownership' in the case of a post-mortem. For example, talking to parents about when they are 'allowed' to see their child denies their *right* to do so.

Practical examples of the kind of information required follow.

Legalities

Usually a doctor (but sometimes a nurse with an extended role) will confirm the death. The death must be reported to the coroner who will decide whether a post-mortem examination is necessary or that the doctor may issue a certificate as to the medical cause of death. Assuming that the doctor is able to issue a certificate, the death is then registered with the registrar for births, marriages and deaths, by either or both parents, whether married or not. In extreme circumstances, someone else present at the death or during the last illness can do this. In the case of a newly born baby, the birth can be declared at the same time as the death is registered. The registrar issues:

➤ the death certificate, for which a small fee is payable
➤ a green disposal form, which is needed by the undertaker to remove the body from hospital, unless a post-mortem is required.

However, the parents are entitled to remove the body themselves once a doctor has confirmed the cause of death. This situation may arise when the child dies after 5 p.m. and the parents are unwilling to leave the child in the hospital mortuary overnight or over the weekend before they can register the death. Parents have the right to know that this option is available to them, however undesirable this course of action may appear.

LSCB functions relating to child deaths

As part of the Laming Report recommendations following the death of Victoria Climbie in 2000, local authorities have set up Local Safeguarding Children Boards (LSCBs). These are made up of strategic heads of service including police, health, education and social care, and are responsible for setting up a Child Death Review Panel. This panel is required by law to consider **all** child deaths in the area, with the following functions:

- collecting and analysing information about the death
- identifying any matter of concern affecting the safety and welfare of children, including any case needing a serious case review
- identifying any general public health or safety concerns arising
- putting in place procedures for ensuring a coordinated response by the authority to an unexpected death of a child.

(*Working Together to Safeguard Children*, Department for Children, Schools and Families, 2006.)

In cases of sudden death or where the cause of death is not known

The doctor must inform the coroner. In most coroners' jurisdictions, when the death is sudden and unexpected a SUDI protocol will determine the engagement and actions of the professionals who will investigate the death. Usually a doctor and a police officer acting on behalf of the coroner will interview the parents. A post-mortem examination is normally required and an inquest may follow to determine how, when and where the child died. An inquest may be necessary either because the death of the child may be due to unnatural causes or because the pathologist is not able immediately to determine the cause of death without further tests.

Once a medical cause of death is established or the inquest has been concluded, as the case may be, the death can be registered and the body released. In the case of a coroner's post-mortem, the coroner sends a certificate as to the cause of death to the registrar of births, deaths and marriages to enable the parents to register the death. In the case of an inquest, the coroner registers the death on the conclusion of the inquest. If no inquest is required, however, the parents are given leave to register the death. Parents should be asked if they want to know what the post-mortem examination entails. Many do not like to ask, but are later filled with remorse for not knowing, and may suffer from fantasies of butchery. Reassurance of standard procedures and sensitive handling of the body are welcome.

In cases where a post-mortem is not legally required, it may still be requested for the sake of medical research, and is then a matter of choice. Post-mortems may be problematic for Muslims, Jews and Hindus unless ordered by the coroner.

Access to the child's body

It is essential that the parents are given privacy to spend as long as they wish with the child after death in hospital. It is helpful for one of the nursing staff to prepare them for the changes that will occur in the temperature and appearance of the body. They should be invited to take part in the washing and dressing of the child's body and other laying-out procedures, but should not be pressed to do so. Practising Muslim, Hindu and Jewish families are responsible for attending to the body to carry out traditional post-death rituals.

The taking of a photograph or lock of hair is now routinely offered by most hospitals, although the family's permission must be obtained: it is important to Muslims that the hair is not cut after death.

Parents are often very anxious to know where the child's body is taken after they have said their goodbyes. Again, they often do not like to ask: they are swept along in a personal nightmare and feel constrained by institutional procedures. They need to be told exactly what will happen to the child, where the body will be kept, who will tend to it and when they are able to visit. Ideally an 'open access' policy enables parents to come back to the hospital and spend time with their child at any hour of the day or night.

Options for where the child rests before the funeral

It is incumbent on professionals to make parents aware of the options, as some parents do not realise that they can have their child's body at home for some or all of the time before the funeral. Those families who have exercised this option have found it very beneficial. Again, it is a question of giving control back where it belongs.

Burial or cremation?

Parents naturally shrink from the thought of either burying or burning their child's body. Muslims are always buried, never cremated. All adult Hindus are cremated, but infants and young children may be buried. Orthodox Jews are always buried, but those of a more liberal persuasion may choose cremation. Where religious faith allows a choice, parents may welcome talking through the pros and cons with an objective outsider before making such an irrevocable decision. This means allowing time for making informed decisions.

Having a specific place to visit is an important consideration for most families. An unforeseen dilemma can later occur when a grandparent or other relative generously offers to open an existing family grave so that the baby or child is not 'alone'. This may be an attractive idea at the time, but can be later regretted with the realisation that the parents are then unable to join their child after death, as they would if they had opened a new family grave. These are Lisa's reflections:

> 'I was in such a daze after Carl died, but I knew I didn't want him buried. I couldn't have coped with the thought of his little body under the ground. There's a special garden of remembrance in our town where the ashes of babies can be scattered, so that's what we did. It seemed a nice idea to have him with other children. But I wish someone had told us that we could have bought a special little plot there. When we visit, I envy other parents who can plant flowers and have a little plaque to sit by.
>
> Another thing I realised too late, after talking to other mums, was that I could have had Carl home before the funeral.
>
> They were very good at the hospital and let us visit him, and then we went to see him at the chapel of rest, but it was never long enough. I'd have liked him home for at least a couple of days.'

Funeral expenses

Funeral costs vary and it is advisable to obtain more than one quotation. Some funeral directors deliver a free basic service for any child who dies under the age of 16. Parents who can ill afford a funeral may reject this as charity, and need reassurance that a free service is of equal quality and is likely to indicate a particular sensitivity to child death situations. The hospital has an obligation to arrange and pay for the funeral of stillborn children, whether born in hospital or at home.

Families receiving Income Support or some other DSS benefits are entitled to help with some or all of the funeral costs, and with the cost of transporting the body within the UK if the child dies away from home.

ATTENDING THE FUNERAL

The funeral presents a ritual opportunity for family and community to say final goodbyes, and for others to pay their respects to the grieving family.

The advisability of young children attending funerals

Parents often consult professionals about whether their young children should go to the funeral. This is really a question of what adults can tolerate. Any temptation to tell parents what to do should be resisted. It is much more helpful to explore with them the pros and cons, to offer points of view they may not have considered, and encourage them to trust their own judgement. When parents are caught between their own instincts to take the children and the disapproving voices of older relatives, the task is one of reassurance.

Most children who were denied the opportunity to attend a sibling's funeral later regret this. Those who would not have wished to go regret not being given the choice. The age at which children can be trusted with such a choice will depend on the degree of openness in the family.

It is more of a dilemma for the professional when it is obvious that the parents have simply assumed that children should not attend funerals and have not considered the possible benefits of taking them. Should the parents' unconsidered judgement be challenged, or is this professional interference? The use of open questions is helpful here, for example:

➤ 'Have you thought about other options?'
➤ 'What has led you to make this decision?'

Professionals attending funerals

The public part of the funeral is the proper place for all affected by the death of the child to share their grief. Nurses, teachers, social workers, health visitors and doctors who have been closely involved with the child and family may wish to attend on their own behalf, or to represent their agency. Either way, it means a lot to the family to know that they were there. Rotas may limit the numbers of staff who can go, but managers who recognise the importance of key staff attending this ritual will try to accommodate their requests.

ON FIRST VISITING THE FAMILY

With or without previous knowledge of the family, the first visit to the home after the bereavement is fraught with anxiety. Typical concerns are:

➤ will the family welcome my visit?
➤ is it the right time to go?
➤ what can I say?
➤ will I be overwhelmed by their grief?

There is no magic formula to dispel the apprehension, but self-preparation can help to prevent unnecessary stress. Many of the following points relate to common sense and common good practice, but in the context of heightened emotions they can easily be forgotten.

Be realistic

Part of the anxiety comes from believing that you have to know the right thing to say that will help to ease their pain, so it is immediately freeing to acknowledge to yourself what an unrealistic expectation this is. Nothing you can say or do will help to bring back the life of the child, which would be the only thing to make the family 'feel better' at this time. You are guaranteed to feel helpless as a result.

Be realistic about the amount of follow-up support you can offer, so that you do not end up promising more than you can maintain.

Be prepared

It helps to double-check the information you have about the family, in particular the name and age of the child. Allow for more time than you might generally give to a home visit. If this is the first time you have been involved with the family, or when the death is sudden, it is likely that the full story needs to be told. To do justice to the child's memory and the parents' feelings, the story should not be rushed. Learning how to end your visit and when to withdraw is a skill that comes with experience! It is made easier if you say at the beginning what time is available to you. It is useful to remember that your visit will be emotionally draining for the family as well as for you. If you can, arrange your timetable so that you allow for the impact on you, by setting aside time afterwards to debrief with a colleague.

Be clear

Introduce yourself and say who you are representing. If you are not expected, check whether your visit at this time is convenient. The purpose of your visit may be obvious to you, but at a time of such confusion it is important to say what it is. In the first few days, the family may be visited by many different professionals and befrienders. It is helpful if you leave details of your name, organisation, contact number and availability. Make it clear whether you will visit again, and if so, when that will be. An unscheduled visit from the GP or clergy can leave the family with unrealistic expectations of future visits which turn to disappointment. It is a good idea to follow up your first contact with a telephone call or a note if no other arrangement was made on your departure.

Be honest and genuine

The general principles detailed in Chapter 4 are all relevant, none more so than the warning against platitudes, which have a nasty habit of slipping out at times of anxiety. Nerves can also lead to inappropriate trading of your own experience, which should be firmly resisted, especially on this first visit. Bland reassurances do not comfort. A parent recalls the words of a visiting priest: 'You must remember that God's only son suffered on the cross for us.' The parent replied: 'Yes, but he didn't suffer for 18 months, like my son.'

If you feel lost for words, it does no harm to say so. A touch of the hand can say far more than words. Accepting periods of silence and displays of emotion may be the most difficult but most valuable gift you can offer.

ANNIVERSARIES

Anniversaries are powerful replays of events and the emotions that accompanied them. Many parents find that the anticipation of the anniversary, during the preceding days, is as bad or worse than the day itself. Significant anniversaries also include the 'might-have-been' birthdays or other celebrations, as well as turning points in the terminal illness or events leading up to the death.

A contact of some kind by carers at the time of the anniversary of the death – particularly the first – is very much valued by the family, whether or not active support is ongoing. Many bereavement support organisations recommend a minimum of 13 months' support in order to help the bereaved through the first anniversary. The contact that is made, by card, letter, telephone or visit, should always refer to the child by name. For example, the simplest wording on a card might be: 'To Andrew's family, with kind thoughts at this special time'.

If you are in regular contact with the family, do not be afraid of talking about the anniversary beforehand. Your support may be helpful in thinking through their options for marking the occasion, or in working out strategies for simply getting through the day.

For those who fantasise about rejoining their loved ones, the anniversary of the death may focus any suicidal thoughts. If your relationship with the parents allows, it is better to confront such thoughts than avoid them – *see* below.

SUICIDE RISK ASSESSMENT

Suicidal thoughts are common to bereaved parents, particularly in the first year of bereavement, and can be anticipated as normal. Contrary to public myth, you cannot put such ideas into people's heads by mentioning them. Fears of self-harm are generally diluted by talking about them and having them acknowledged. Although it is dangerous to generalise, the following pointers may help you to assess the risk of actual self-harm.

Usually a statement or implication of suicidal intent is concerned with ending one's misery rather than one's life. Typical comments are:

➤ 'I want to be with him and hold him again.'
➤ 'I want to go to bed and not wake up again.'
➤ 'Life is meaningless without him.'
➤ 'I can't go on like this.'
➤ 'He needs me more than the rest of the family.'

Any such remark needs an acknowledgement that you have heard the desperate feelings conveyed. An appropriate response might be:

'You sound as if you don't want to go on living – is that so?'

If the reply is affirmative, the next step is to ask whether that means a conscious wish to die:

'Do you mean you want to end your life?'

This feels very risky, but be assured that in nearly all cases this question will draw a conditional response, such as:

'Yes, I think about it, but I wouldn't do anything because . . .'

Now you can relax a little, and safely invite further exploration of how those awful feelings are experienced, and try to convey some understanding of their validity. But what if your question draws a different response?

'Yes, I've thought it all out.'

Or, simply, 'Yes.'

In this situation, the alarm bells are now ringing. Having gone so far, you need to follow with a question that will give a clear indication of purpose:

'Have you thought what you would do?'

Do not be afraid of asking this question, as it is key to the assessment of risk. The response may again be conditional:

'Well, I've thought of crashing the car, but I couldn't bear to hurt the rest of the family even more.'

Now you are dealing with some intent, balanced with reservations, which can be strengthened with your support. However, the response may be more specific:

'Oh yes. I have got the pills all saved up, and I know exactly how many to take.'

Such a detailed method needs to be taken as a serious statement of intent. This is rare, but if you are faced with this situation, *you must seek support and advice*. The ethical question of whether you should take any action without this person's consent needs to be considered. If you conclude that you should alert someone else with your worries, you must inform the person you are supporting that you are doing so out of concern for their safety and welfare.

Again, the need for good support and supervision for yourself is underlined by any doubts you may have on this score.

Following a suicide

It is truly shocking and distressing to contemplate a young person choosing to end his or her own life. Following the death of a young person by his or her own hand, parents and schools alike will be understandably anxious about the effect on other vulnerable children and how to prevent 'copycat' self-harming behaviours. For some guidance in this stressful situation, *see* Chapter 8, *Support for schools*, pp 177–9.

Reference

Department for Children, Schools and Families. *Working Together to Safeguard Children.* London: HM Government; 2006.

Further reading

Buckman R. *How to Break Bad News: a guide for healthcare professionals.* London: Papermac; 1992.

CHAPTER 6

Guidelines for talking with children

'Sorrow makes us all children again.'

Ralph Waldo Emerson

INTRODUCTION

This is an area that understandably causes a lot of anxiety. What to say, and how to say it, are the two big questions for parents and teachers facing the task of informing siblings and peers of a child who is dying, or has died. Medical personnel will also face these dilemmas, alongside the parents, with the child who is terminally ill. It goes against the grain to expose children to the harsh reality of another child's death, when the instinct is to protect them from pain. Talking to children about death also exposes adults to feelings of helplessness and uncertainty, making them vulnerable to questions that may have no answers.

What we do know is that children suffer more from ignorance than honesty, and that children are surprisingly resilient given a supportive environment.

While anxieties centre on what to tell children, the first move may come from the child asking for information, usually when the adult is least prepared! Either way, the desired outcome is a dialogue between adult and child, which involves as much listening as talking. Talking *to* children becomes talking *with* children.

In situations where the child's needs indicate special attention, it is important not to make the child feel more different and isolated than she already feels as a result of her experience. Involve her family, peers, or other trusted adults as far as possible.

The guidelines offered here are based on general principles and may be applied to most situations. In extreme cases, when the child has been exposed to severe trauma, referral to a specialist should be considered.

Readers of this chapter should also refer to Chapter 2, pp 48–50, regarding the development of children's understanding of death, and to Chapter 8.

Further advice for parents is offered in Chapter 7, pp 158–60.

CHILD EXPERIENCE OF LOSS AND BEREAVEMENT

Although child and adult experiences of grief are different, children are people and children do grieve, even very young children. Their understanding of loss and death will obviously vary according to age and ability, so that explanations need to be age-appropriate.

Young children under five see death as temporary, and need repeated confirmation that the dead child will not be coming back. Up to age six or seven, children go through a stage of 'magical thinking' when they don't yet know the limits to the power of their own thoughts and wishes. Thus, they are particularly vulnerable to feelings of guilt and responsibility for the death, however irrational that may seem to an adult. Even very young children can be sensitive to their parents' distress and learn not to talk about their own anxieties.

Children between six and 10 become aware of the reality of death, gradually developing an understanding that dead means 'can't breathe, can't move, can't feel', and that death is universal and inevitable. Although they are more aware, they may not understand the feelings they are experiencing or associate them with their loss and may become distressed as a result. Thus, a child who is not yet emotionally mature enough to talk about feelings may 'act out' her grief through aggressive behaviour or disturbed sleep.

From the age of 11 children begin to develop a more adult concept of death, and may learn to cope with the awareness of their own mortality through black humour and bravado.

An important aspect of bereavement for children is the *secondary losses* that follow from the loss of the child who has died (Hindmarch, 1995). So, for example, a child may be affected more by losing the attention of a grieving parent than by the death of a baby brother she never knew. Loss of security, trust and normality following the death of a sibling or friend may have implications reaching far beyond the immediate loss of their physical presence and companionship.

The biggest issues for children, as reported by children themselves, sometimes long after the event, are to do with *information* and *involvement*. Children who seem to cope best are those who are kept informed about what is happening, are told about the death in unambiguous terms, and are involved in rituals such as the funeral. Children who are protected from the truth and excluded from the rest of the family, for example by being sent away to relatives or back to school at the time of the funeral, are likely to become bewildered, frightened or resentful. Children make up what they don't know, and their imaginings are usually worse than the truth. Silence to a child may well feed the fantasy that she is to blame for the death. Silence will certainly risk a loss of trust between adult and child.

It is, of course, impossible not to communicate with children. They are adept at picking up atmospheres and feelings, and they will instinctively understand if the adults around them do not want to talk or show their feelings. Adults often assume it is they who are protecting children from anxieties, when it is children who protect adults from the upset, which feels more frightening when shrouded in mystery. So what do children need to help address their anxieties?

The most common anxieties experienced by children relate to:

➤ *responsibility*: Was it my fault? Did I somehow cause the death? Could I have done anything to stop it happening? Why him and not me?
➤ *mortality*: Will I die too? Am I at risk? Will it be my turn next? Who else will die?
➤ *security*: Who will look out for me now? How will I keep safe? What will happen? Am I still loved and accepted?

Such concerns may be verbalised, though more commonly they are expressed in physical and behavioural reactions, particularly in younger children. These may include:

➤ anxiety about being separated from parents or carers
➤ difficulty in going to sleep, or fear of the dark
➤ regressing to an earlier stage, such as clinging, bedwetting or baby talk
➤ a tendency to infections
➤ reluctance to go to school
➤ difficulty in concentrating
➤ over-eating, or conversely losing interest in food

- ➤ developing a phobia about doctors or hospitals
- ➤ angry and aggressive outbursts
- ➤ becoming withdrawn and depressed.

These are normal reactions and most will pass with time. Meanwhile there are some practical responses that can be put in place, such as providing a nightlight, but in general the overwhelming need is for understanding and reassurance. At a time of bewilderment and upheaval, the child needs to be held emotionally and perhaps physically too.

FIRST PRINCIPLES

These are becoming clear from the above consideration of what we observe and what children themselves report of their bereavement experiences. So far we have identified the common needs of children for:
- ➤ information and explanation about the illness, death, funeral etc
- ➤ inclusion and involvement in discussions, plans, decisions, rituals
- ➤ understanding and reassurance about their feelings and concerns.

It follows that the adults seeking to meet these needs require a level of openness, warmth and honesty in communicating with children. It may also take courage.

Who is best placed to talk with the child?

Obviously the parents are ideally suited to meet the needs and conditions listed above. When that is not possible, it should be a known and trusted adult, who has an ongoing relationship with the child.

Other family members or close friends may help out if the parent is in extreme distress. Parents who are in shock, or absorbed with practical tasks around the time of the death, may need some prompting and guidance from concerned professionals: 'Have you thought what you are going to say to his sister?' Later, it is helpful for parents and teachers to discuss what the child has been told and how the death is experienced or understood within the family's culture and belief systems.

When to talk?

The simple answer is, as soon as possible. When it comes to giving bad news or information about the death, any delay makes it more likely that the child will be told by the wrong person in an unhelpful way. The child has to know eventually and may misinterpret any delay or avoidance as indicating some fault or blame attached to herself. At the very least, delay suggests disinterest, and risks isolating the child from the rest of the family.

Timing is not so obvious when the adult is concerned to give the child an opportunity to express and explore her reactions and to open up a dialogue. Then it may be better to make spaces and times that encourage open communication, such as bathtime, bedtime, storytime, walking the dog together, asking for help with a task.

Familiarity with the child and sensitivity to her temperament will then determine whether it is better to initiate the dialogue, or offer some cues to signal your willingness to listen, or simply wait for the child to talk when ready.

How to communicate with children and young people

In his introduction to his book *Talking About Death*, Earl Grollman offers this advice:

> 'Approach the discussion gently and lovingly; the tone of your voice should be warm, sympathetic, kind. *What* is said is significant, but *how* you say it will have a greater bearing on whether youngsters develop morbid fears or will be able to accept, within their capacity, the reality of death.'

Grollman also reminds us to go at the child's pace. Young children particularly need time to absorb information and time to come back to their feelings and queries, perhaps after some distracting play between.

The following guidelines on communicating with children build on the experience of Barbara Monroe at St Christopher's Hospice and other people working with bereaved children and families.

➤ *Talk at eye level.* This is fundamental. It signals interest and a willingness to engage in a real dialogue with the child. It creates the right conditions for reading body language, picking up clues, and responding in a respectful way. It facilitates touching and holding (if appropriate). It is non-threatening and non-patronising.

➤ *Speak directly to and with the child.* This may seem obvious, but at stressful times it's all too easy for adults – particularly professionals – to speak to the child through another adult.

➤ *Avoid confusing and ambivalent language.* Examples are legion and legendary: 'We have lost your brother/He has gone to sleep forever/ He has passed away.' The corollary advice is not to be afraid to use the words 'death', 'dying' and 'dead'.

➤ *Avoid clichés and platitudes.* These readily spring to the lips when anxious to protect or reassure the child: 'Perhaps it's for the best/The good die young.' Such phrases are no help to the child and only serve to protect the adult from the discomfort of facing reality.

➤ *Keep explanations short and simple.* Be prepared to repeat explanations, perhaps in different ways. Link observations to what the child already knows and what she has experienced. Ask what she thinks and feels. Use the images she offers.

➤ *Check the child's understanding.* Grollman tells a lovely story of how we need to check that the meaning of the speaker meets the understanding of the listener:

> 'I was once asked by a young girl, "How long is death?" I responded, "Death is permanent." The youngster said, "Oh, then it's not so bad." Noticing my bewilderment she said simply, "My mother has permanents at the hairdresser. It doesn't last very long". (Grollman, 1990)

Even simple words can be misunderstood. A friend of mine grasped the nettle when her little boy asked what had happened to his friend after he had died. She explained how the body was washed and dressed; how the body would be placed in the coffin; and even what would happen to the body after burial. His puzzled look was explained by his next question: 'And what happens to the head?'

➤ *Be truthful and honest.* The cost of hiding or avoiding the truth is to lose the trust of the child. Children are amazingly resilient and often surprise us by their ability to handle difficult information. There is a caveat to this guideline, of course, which is to use language appropriate to the child's age and ability. Being honest may involve answering difficult questions with 'I don't know' or 'I'm not sure' or 'I'll come back to you on that when I've had time to think'. Honesty may also mean owning your feelings: 'I am hurt/angry/puzzled too.'

➤ *Keep them informed.* Tell the child what has happened/is happening and what will happen next. Prepare her for changes in others and herself.

➤ *Keep the dialogue open.* This does not mean pushing the child to talk, but being aware of the child's need to revisit their reactions to the death in the future, as well as the special effect of anniversaries and significant life changes.

Finally, remember that there are more questions than answers. It is more important to listen to a child's concerns and to show you have heard them, than to meet questions with 'right' answers.

HELPING CHILDREN UNDERSTAND ABOUT TERMINAL ILLNESS

Children who have lived with a sibling's chronic illness will be used to the stresses and strains that it brings for all family members. They may experience frequent separations from the sick sibling when hospitalised and indeed from parents. Inevitably parents have less time and energy to spend with their well children, and daily routines are disrupted. Well children may not, however, understand that the illness is life-threatening, or that the ill child will die (even when the outcome is obvious to the adult) unless they are prepared. Preparation is also needed for changes in the sick child's condition and whatever consequences may follow.

What about the direct question, 'Is he going to die?' Anticipating such a question, perhaps with the support of another adult, can help the parent or professional prepare a response that manages to balance realism with hope, such as, 'I hope he won't die, but he is very poorly, and the doctor says he might not get better.'

Children are helped by the adults around them talking to each other. There are obvious benefits to children in maintaining school routines and out-of-school activities, and when teachers and club leaders are kept informed of what is happening in the family, they can respond in a helpful way.

Teenagers are particularly vulnerable as they get caught up in the ambivalent feelings of adolescence. They may swing from wanting to take on an adult helping role, to being resentful of disruption to their normal life. Teenagers may be less likely to initiate discussion with adults, turning more naturally to friends, but they are still in need of up-to-date information and the opportunities to talk. Some find that talking is easier with teachers, doctors and nurses than with parents.

INFORMING CHILDREN OF THE DEATH

Faced with such a difficult task, you may need to deal with your own anxieties first. Talking it through with a friend or colleague can help to clarify what needs to be said and what may get in the way of saying it. Apart from any practical problems regarding the time and place, it will be your feelings which will cause concern: embarrassment; fear of the child's distress; fear of becoming upset yourself; wanting to get it right; and feeling clumsy and helpless. Naming and facing those feelings can go a good way towards reducing their impact.

As part of your preparation you may find it useful to rehearse what you are going to say, either verbally or in writing. How this is done will depend on the situation.

➤ In one-to-one meetings with a child, you can access *more* spontaneity and sincerity by having considered the options beforehand and then putting them out of your mind, trusting to the moment.

➤ In situations where your task is to address a group of children, you are well advised to have a crib sheet of the points you want to cover, to ensure they are not lost as the interactive group process unfolds.

➤ If several adults are going to speak to several groups concurrently, as may happen in larger schools, it makes sense for a prepared script to be available. This ensures consistency, that the same information is received by different groups. It also helps those who are feeling diffident and ill-equipped, as the script can be read or adapted to the individual's style. Some schools that have faced this situation have put in extra helpers, such as volunteer parents or classroom assistants, to support or share the teacher's task.

A prepared script might go something like this:

'I want you all to listen carefully as I have some very sad news to tell you, which might upset you. Some of you may already have heard that Jan was knocked down by a car yesterday evening while he was out on his bike. He was badly injured and was taken to hospital. He had an operation and the doctors tried very hard to save his life. Sadly he was too badly hurt to recover, and he died in the early hours of this morning. His mum and dad have sent a message to say that they are not sure how it happened, but they think Jan lost control of his bike coming down the hill near his house, and swerved into the path of a car which couldn't stop in time. Jan was knocked out and did not regain consciousness, so, although he was badly injured, he didn't feel any pain. That's all we know at the moment. Later there will be a public report called an inquest, which will investigate how and why he died. There will be a funeral some time next week, and Jan's family would like the school to be involved somehow. I will let you know as soon as the school has further information about that.'

Such a script offers a form of words which may be used, but more importantly it covers the essential elements for enabling the expression of grief:
➤ what happened
➤ how it happened
➤ why it happened
➤ what happens next.

These components help the child confront the reality of the death and begin to try and make some sense of it. A base has been established for the expression of the child's reactions and the asking of questions, and time needs to be made available for this. Children of all ages, and particularly younger children, welcome the opportunity to move on to practical tasks and plans to focus their energy, such as a card, collage, poem, memory corner or website.

In summary, a checklist of breaking sad news to children follows the same principles as the guidelines on breaking bad news at the beginning of Chapter 5.

➤ **Why?**   Because otherwise the child will get to know in less desirable ways.

             To engender trust and to facilitate the healthy expression of grief.

➤ **When?**   As soon as possible.

➤ **By whom?** By someone known and trusted by the child(ren).

➤ **Where?**   In familiar, safe and comfortable surroundings.

➤ **How?**   In a straightforward and unambiguous way, in language that is easily understood, with sensitivity, with time and opportunity to express feelings and ask questions.

Finally, get support for yourself. It is just as important to have the support of that friend or colleague afterwards to pick up on how it went and how you are left feeling.

TELLING CHILDREN ABOUT A MURDER OR SUICIDE

> 'I knew she was missing but they didn't tell me anything else . . . the way I found out she was murdered was from the television. It was like they couldn't be bothered to tell me.'

It is easy to understand the bewilderment and hurt of this young teenager whose older sister was murdered. But imagine also the shocked state of her parents at the time, unable to bring themselves to tell their younger daughter what they did not want to believe themselves. It's easy with hindsight to see the folly of trying to protect her from the truth for as long as possible. Even a few minutes' reflection will show up the blind spot in this logic. Of course the surviving siblings, and other children, will get to know the circumstances of the death, sooner or later, from children in the playground, from overhearing adults or through the media. And the more sensational the cause of death, notably murder or suicide, the more likely it is that rumour and fantasy will distort the truth. Another few minutes' reflection serves to remind us that when children learn that they were not told the truth, they are commonly led to one of two conclusions: that they cannot trust those adults in the future; or that they must somehow be to blame, and that's why they were not told.

It's hard enough for us as adults to come to terms with such destructive acts as the murder or suicide of a child without the added burden of telling other children. So here again the starting point is to pay attention to your own reactions, even if you have to put them on hold for the time being while you address immediate tasks. Give yourself some breathing space to discuss with a colleague, or consult with a specialist, how you are going to tackle this delicate subject with the child(ren) in your care.

Younger children may well need help with understanding new words such as murder, manslaughter, homicide, suicide, overdose etc. The more difficult task is to help them with the concepts behind the words. How can we understand the murder of a child, or the self-destructive act of a young person?

A second but separate issue is how much detail to include in the telling. Is it (a) necessary and (b) appropriate to say how the young person was murdered or how he took his own life? If you had the task of communicating such news to primary school classes, what would you say to Year Six children that you wouldn't say to Year One children (who may have siblings in Year Six)?

Again, there are more questions than answers, and each one needs careful consideration. These are also times for trusting that your own sincerity and compassion will be understood and respected by even very young children, even when you are struggling for words.

The following vignettes are offered for consideration, one the murder of a seven-year-old girl, and the other the suicide of a 16-year-old boy. Both are based on true stories but hopefully disguised beyond recognition.

Esther's murder

Esther, aged seven, went missing on a Thursday and on Saturday her naked body was found on waste ground a mile from her home. A post-mortem held on Sunday revealed that she had been sexually assaulted and had died from head injuries. The same day a young man was arrested and charged with her murder.

The headteacher of the school attended by Esther and her five-year-old sister faced the dilemma of what to say to the children on Monday. The night before she consulted with her deputy, the police, the chair of governors, Esther's parents, and other parents. She decided to use the same form of words with each class in turn:

'I have something to say to you which is very sad and hard to understand. Some of you know that Esther was missing last Thursday and no-one could find her. Everyone was very worried.

I went to see her mother and father on Friday, and they were upset because they did not know what had happened or where she was. Then on Saturday a policeman came to see me and told me that something really bad had happened to Esther. A woman walking her dog found Esther lying in some long grass. But she wasn't moving or breathing because she was dead. The police took her body to the hospital for some tests. The tests showed that Esther had died because someone had killed her. This is called murder. Esther had been injured/hurt in different parts of her body, but the injuries to her head were the ones which killed her. That means we can hope she died quickly and didn't feel much hurt.

The police think they have caught the man who did this to Esther, but they don't know for sure. They will keep this man in prison until the case comes to court in a few months' time, so we don't have to worry about that.

It's hard to understand why anyone should want to hurt and kill Esther. Some people say that this man must be bad, and some say he must be mad. It's rare for a murder to happen. Most people grow old without knowing anyone who has been murdered but they might read about it in the paper or hear about it on the news.'

What would *you* have said?

Jordan's suicide

At the age of 16 Jordan rarely attended school and supported his increasing drug use with odd jobs and petty theft. In spite of a bravado exterior, he experienced black moods. His relationship with his parents was stormy and he frequently 'left home' to stay with other family members. So a note he left for his mum after the last argument saying 'I am going for good this time' was not taken too seriously. When he was found hanged in a disused barn it seemed impossible to draw any other conclusion than that he intended to take his own life. The post-mortem showed a cocktail of drugs present in his body, including hallucinogenic substances.

After consultation, the headteacher scripted the following statement for form tutors:

'This is a very sad day for the school. Many of you will have heard the tragic news of Jordan's death. I want to tell you what happened, with the agreement of Jordan's family, to avoid rumour and speculation. We know how he died. We know that he hanged himself, which means he probably died instantly. We don't know why he died. As you know, when someone ends their own life, this is called suicide. It's very difficult to understand why anyone should want to kill themselves. It's rare, and it usually happens when someone is extremely confused or depressed, much worse than the normal feelings of being mixed up or fed up that most people have from time to time. We do know that Jordan was under the influence of drugs when he died, but we don't know how much the drugs affected his state of mind. It's important not to guess or make assumptions, even if we knew Jordan well. It is the job of the inquest, which is an official enquiry, to look at all the evidence as to how and why Jordan died.'

Would you phrase this differently? What else would you say?

(*See* also the end of Chapter 8, *Support for schools*, 'After a suicide'.)

SUMMARY OF DOS AND DON'TS

➤ **Do** aim for dialogue, rather than talking at children.
➤ **Do** practise using the 'death' word and talking about death as a fact of life.
➤ **Do** remember the importance of information and involvement for children.
➤ **Do** prepare yourself and what you are going to say.
➤ **Do** allow for a child's expression of grief, and for a child's questions.
➤ **Do** allow yourself to show your feelings.
➤ **Do** seek consultation and support for yourself.
➤ **Don't** use stories and fairy tales to explain the mystery of death.
➤ **Don't** make out that you have all the answers.
➤ **Don't** leave room for a child's wondering whether she might have been to blame.
➤ **Don't** underestimate your ability to help a child by listening and showing you care.

References

Grollman EA. *Talking About Death: a dialogue between parent and child.* Boston: Beacon Press; 1990.

Hindmarch C. Secondary losses for siblings. *Child Care Health Dev.* 1995; **21**(6): 425–31.

Yule W, Gold A. *Wise Before the Event.* London: Calouste Gulbenkian Foundation; 1993.

Further reading

Turner M. *Talking with Children and Young People about Death and Dying.* London: Jessica Kingsley Publishers; 1998.

Stokes JA, Crossley D. *Beyond the Rough Rock: supporting a child who is bereaved through suicide.* Cheltenham: Winston's Wish; 2001 (last updated April 2008). (*See* Appendix A for Winston's Wish contact details.)

SECTION 3

Bereavement support

CHAPTER 7

Support for families

'Hope is incredible to the prisoner of grief.'

Petrarch

The kind of support offered should ideally be determined by the needs of the bereaved, but realistically it will also depend on what resources are available. Different models for support services will be considered in Chapter 9, but first it is necessary to describe the various approaches and what they aim to achieve. Other questions addressed are:

➤ how and when is this strategy appropriate?
➤ who offers this kind of help?
➤ how can this support be obtained?

PRACTICAL SUPPORT

In the early days there is usually a need for practical support, particularly in the case of sudden death. Parents in extreme shock may find themselves unable to care adequately for their other children. They may find it hard to sleep, or to think about food, or to apply themselves to the practical arrangements that need to be made. The offer of a lift or childminding or the gift of a casserole can convey as much comfort as any words.

Ideally this kind of practical help is forthcoming from extended family, friends and neighbours who are sensitive to the parents' needs. However, not all parents want relief from practical tasks and would prefer to be busy doing things as a way of coping with the pain. It needs to be their choice. If in doubt, ask them. There is no virtue in guessing, although there is often an expectation that one should know what is best for other people!

Well-meaning relatives may be overzealous in their concern to protect their loved ones. An obvious example is the tendency for brothers and sisters of the dying or dead child being bundled away from the scene of action. Even at a very young age children will experience a sense of exclusion if they are 'sent away' at such a time.

They may then feel somehow punished and guilty, but are likely to comply with the expectations of the adults around them that they should play nicely and not ask questions. Children learn quickly to protect their protectors. On the other hand, some children may be very relieved to have some respite from distress, and welcome the chance to stay with a favourite aunt for a break.

How does one know which course is preferred by a particular child? Ask the child. Even very young children, once freed of responsibility for 'looking after' their parents, know what they want and can be trusted to know what is right for them. If the possible alternatives are openly offered, for example 'Do you want to stay here with Mummy and Daddy tonight, or do you want to stay the night with Granny?', most children will give a truthful answer. As well as getting it right for the child, it is equally important to the child that she has been asked.

An example of well-meaning relatives not taking account of a parent's wishes is given here by Joyce:

> 'I was 19 and unmarried when I had my first baby, and that was seen as a disgrace in those days. It was the year of the Aberfan tragedy. Catherine was born with the cord round her neck and she only lived 10 minutes. Somebody said: "It's the best thing that could have happened". There were complications so I had to stay in hospital for two weeks. My mum saw to the funeral and I only found out later where the baby was buried. The worst was when I got home: my mum had given everything away that I'd got ready for the baby – cot, pram, clothes, the lot. I know she thought she was doing it for the best, but I had nothing tangible left to connect with the baby and what I'd lost, nothing to grieve with.'

Not everyone has a good network of family support to fall back on.

When this is the case, key community figures such as the clergy, church visitor or social worker will assume more significance in providing practical help. Where several people are involved it is obviously important to co-ordinate efforts and to work cooperatively. The family doctor might most naturally take on this co-ordinating role, although it could just as easily be the health visitor or social worker.

Whatever the role, any visitor to the home of a bereaved family is likely to feel apprehensive – may actually be terrified – about the level of distress within, and conscious of not knowing what to say or do to help. It takes courage to make the first call. However, having made contact, it is important only to offer support that can realistically be maintained.

BEFRIENDING

Several of the specialist support organisations, such as the Foundation for the Study of Infant Deaths, the Scottish Cot Death Trust, and The Compassionate Friends provide a valuable befriending service. More generally, Samaritans may offer face-to-face contact as well as 24-hour crisis support by telephone. Hospices and church visitor schemes, and victim support organisations may also offer a befriending service.

Befriending is rather like a one-way friendship. The helper offers the acceptance and listening ear of a friend without the emotional ties that require mutuality. Talking has many therapeutic effects:

➤ it helps to accept the reality of the loss
➤ it is a way of expressing and discharging emotions
➤ it helps to normalise reactions
➤ it re-establishes order to a disorganised mind.

Most bereaved parents experience the need to go over and over the events surrounding the death and to talk about the baby or child in every detail. This can become wearying for relatives and friends.

Not everyone is as fortunate as Rose:

> 'My sister and brother-in-law visited every evening from the day Paul was killed in September to Christmas. It was the highlight of my day, knowing that Betty was coming round and I could just be myself and talk about Paul.'

Jo and John faced a more usual situation:

'Our families and friends were very supportive at first, but after a few weeks, although people still asked how we were, nobody mentioned *David* any more, when we wanted to talk about him more than ever.'

Having permission and encouragement to talk are crucially important to all bereaved, and the more so when the bereavement is a social embarrassment. Giving that permission and encouragement are key tasks for befrienders. Their value should not be underestimated and this usually voluntary role can be difficult. It demands witnessing another's pain, being faced with unanswerable questions and being left with feelings of helplessness and inadequacy.

Preparation

Ideally the helper will have received some training in listening skills and at least some preparation for the implications of the role.

The conditions of the befriending relationship need to be thought through beforehand regarding availability and expectations. Where does the contact take place? How long should one stay on a home visit? Is a home telephone or mobile number to be given out? The befriender will need support, and should not be left to ask for it if feeling under pressure. A built-in support system is the best way to ensure that the expectations of the role do not become overwhelming.

Who should take on this role?

As in other situations of adversity and trauma, one naturally turns to someone who has suffered a similar experience. There is a common bond that is conducive to trust and understanding. Therefore bereaved parents will often seek out contact with other parents to gain reassurance that they are not alone and that they can survive their tragedy.

If this support is being offered by bereaved parents, they obviously need to have reached the point where they can keep their own grief separate when in this role. Nevertheless, it is likely that their own grief will at times be re-awakened by another's pain, which again underlines the necessity for support.

Whether or not the befriender has lost a child, there is one golden rule: never to say, 'I know exactly how you feel'. This ranks as the cardinal sin of all platitudes. It robs the sufferer of the uniqueness of the individual experience.

When is befriending appropriate?

There is no prescribed time or circumstance, but the following could be taken as indicators:

➤ when the parent is not able to offload to family or friends
➤ when the early support of family and friends has fallen off
➤ when the parent is isolated or housebound
➤ when the parent is struggling with the task of adjustment, practically or emotionally
➤ when the parent is confronting difficult times such as an inquest, birthday, Christmas, anniversary.

Points to consider

➤ Is befriending appropriate?
➤ Is there a suitable helper available?
➤ Are the conditions of the relationship clear?
➤ Is there sufficient support for the befriender?

COUNSELLING

Counselling has taken on a variety of meanings for different people, ranging from advice to long-term therapy. Basic assumptions are that counselling will provide *help* for someone with a *problem*, and that a trained counsellor will have the necessary *skills*. Referrals are often made by other professionals who feel out of their depth and lack the competency required.

It seems important to examine these assumptions in an attempt to clarify the role of the bereavement counsellor and to arrive at some indicators as to when counselling is appropriate.

The purpose of counselling

In many contexts counselling is seen as a problem-solving activity, with the counsellor guiding the client towards resolution of the problem. This idea does not fit comfortably with bereavement, and yet the expectation of both client and referrer is often that the bereavement counsellor will do or say something to make things better. In fact, the focus of the work in all therapeutic counselling is with the client, who sets the pace and the agenda. A more useful view of bereavement counselling is that it provides a means of expressing grief and working on the tasks of mourning. For some, this may be the opportunity to deal with suppressed feelings of anger and despair. For others, bereavement will turn their world upside down in such a way that all areas of life are called into question – relationships, job, religion – and huge adjustments are required. The following comment comes from a staff counsellor:

> 'I have recently had two clients who had lost children through short illnesses. Both of them said that the counselling sessions were like "touching base" in a frightening, changed world, and felt they had benefited from this. I guess they're expressing a sort of "normalising" in an abnormal world.'

The loss of a child questions the meaning of life in a way that few would otherwise face. The loss of a child also contains a very special ingredient: that this child could have been the receiver and giver of the unconditional love we all crave. Thus, the counselling relationship may be instrumental in rebuilding self-esteem and self-worth.

The bereavement counsellor may become, for a while, the ideal parent we all wished we had and would like to be for our children.

Other functions of counselling such as companioning and education may be particularly appropriate to bereavement counselling:

Companioning

Companioning is the name given by Wolfelt (1998) to the kind of counsellor-client relationship well suited to grief work. Basic to this approach is the notion of walking alongside, of being witness to the other's pain and struggle, rather than providing guidance and setting tasks. This model replaces the medical model of treatment, and focuses instead on the change and transformation that come from traumatic loss. It has the merit of empowering the client and normalising grief responses. When 'companioning' is supplemented by agreed interventions as they become needed, it provides a useful format for client-centred bereavement counselling.

Education

An educational component is a feature of a more proactive approach, though it shares with 'companioning' the ideals of empowering the client and of normalising their grief. The educative function is part of a psycho-social approach, to maximise the support available in the community, and to provide information about stress responses as part of a normal process. Arguably this approach helps to reduce the incidence of complicated grieving and prolonged disorders that might require medical intervention later on.

The tasks of counselling

Grief counselling may include any of the following tasks for the mourner:

➤ believing the reality of the loss
➤ experiencing the pain of that loss
➤ understanding one's grief responses
➤ adjusting to daily existence without the loved child
➤ making sense of a world that allowed such a tragic waste
➤ working out one's future direction and reason for living.

This was Barbara's experience:

> 'What brought me to counselling? I just seemed to be caught up in a dense fog which I could not escape from and at times this left me feeling totally lost and almost blind with panic. Counselling helped me to clear the fog and find the sky – even though the sky is still cloudy at times. Counselling has enabled me to sort through my jumbled experiences and feelings and recognise each for what it was. By recognising these things I could deal with those that could be dealt with and learn to live with those that I cannot do anything about. Initially, it helped me to put some perspective into my life. I realised that I was not the only mother to have lost a baby. I directed my thoughts to one issue at a time and gradually I got some sense of control in my life. It has proved to be very liberating.'

The role of the counsellor

It follows from the above that the role of the bereavement counsellor is a demanding one and requires more than the use of counselling skills practised by many other helpers in the course of their work. This distinction is not a judgement of value, nor does it deny the competence of professionals who take on a counselling role without that 'specialist' job title. Indeed, there are many who by nature of their existing professional relationship with the bereaved, such as the GP, health visitor or social worker, are best placed to take it on. However, it is important to be clear about what the role requires and involves. It is misleading and irresponsible when people are described or describe themselves as bereavement counsellors on the basis of goodwill and a day's training in counselling skills. What, then, are the requirements for this role?

➤ Counsellors need to have done sufficient work on their own losses to be aware of their impact on their counselling.

➤ Counsellors need a level of training that has developed understanding of attachment and loss, the features of grief, the tasks of mourning and of the processes at work in the therapeutic relationship.

➤ Counsellors need a setting that gives clear boundaries to the work – a counselling 'contract' – particularly if they have other roles in relation to the client or patient.

➤ Counsellors need supervision to clarify the task in hand and to cope with the emotional demands and feelings of helplessness.

➤ Counsellors need the knowledge and assessment skills required to recognise the relevance of grief reactions to the presentation of depression and anxiety states.

When is counselling appropriate?

As counselling is here defined as more in-depth than listening, more focused and detached than befriending, it follows that it is not appropriate in the early days of grief, not until the first traumatic shock waves from the diagnosis or from the actual death have subsided. It would be the same as starting physiotherapy straight after breaking a leg, instead of allowing time for the initial healing to take place. It may be helpful to pursue this analogy, as not everyone *needs* physiotherapy after breaking a leg. With good health, good healing and good support one can learn to walk again unaided. However, if there are other injuries, if the healing is complicated, or if insufficient attention and time are given to the healing before weight-bearing, it is a different story. Similarly, the painful experience of losing a child may be complicated by particularly traumatic circumstances. It may re-awaken the pain of previous losses, losses that perhaps have not been acknowledged or resolved. Other demands of family or job may not allow time and opportunity to grieve, so that the painful feelings become sup-pressed. In these situations, the focused attention afforded by counselling can help to release the blockages to natural healing.

There are also special features associated with the loss of a child which may complicate grieving and may indicate a need of counselling. One such feature is the fear of insanity, which many parents experience. The frighten-ing and unrelenting extremity of emotions, together with the inability to make sense of what has happened, can send the mind into chaos. Another common experience is feeling suicidal, sometimes driven by guilt, sometimes by a desire to be with the dead baby or child. These reactions are isolating and put a tremendous strain on relationships, between spouses, partners and other family members. The counselling setting can provide a place of safety to discharge these tensions.

As stated above, an early counselling intervention with an educative component may be the most appropriate for those seeking reassurance about their grief responses, and a 'companioning' model is valid for most people. However, counselling is also an obvious resource when chronic grief reactions are manifested in depression, anxiety states, panic attacks and phobic reactions. Family members may present with such symptoms years after the bereavement, and commonly a sensitive GP will make the connection and refer for counselling, perhaps alongside medication.

Counselling, as a talking therapy, offers a safe and structured environment for the client to revisit the traumatic losses underlying their symptoms. The counselling relationship is formalised in a 'contract', i.e. an agreement to work together in clearly defined conditions as to time and place and purpose. Counselling methods will depend on the therapeutic approach favoured by the counsellor, and should also be guided by the client's needs. People who need help in expressing emotions will obviously benefit from a counselling method that focuses on feelings; while those who want to find new meaning and direction in their lives will be better suited to a cognitive approach. The same person may benefit from these different methods at different times, requiring the counsellor to adapt to whatever mode is suitable for the task in hand.

What type of counselling is appropriate?

The movement towards state regulation of counsellors, psychotherapists, and psychological therapists through the Health Professions Council is designed to protect clients and bring more conformity to the type of therapy best suited to relieve symptoms. If seeking counselling through the GP, the counselling approach will be dictated by the medical 'diagnosis', with the emphasis on Cognitive Behavioural Therapy (CBT) as recommended by the National Institute for Health and Clinical Excellence (NICE). According to NICE, CBT is the treatment of choice for depression because it has more measurable outcomes and is structured to give positive results within a short timeframe. This drive for conformity is accompanied by a huge injection of resources by the government to minimise waiting times and to bring consistency to a patchwork of different approaches.

However, these developments reduce access to longer-term, relationship-orientated therapy, they reduce choice of approach and the number of sessions, and they follow a medical model – when most counsellors do not work within a health setting. It is argued elsewhere in this book that there is a real danger in treating grief responses, such as depression, as a disease, and in regarding chronic grief as pathological.

Not everyone can afford a private counsellor, and the choice of practitioner can be bewildering, but arguably the diversity of people seeking counselling support demands an informed choice of various approaches.

Whatever the approach, the common consensus is that the most important ingredient is the *therapeutic relationship* between counsellor and client, which hopefully provides the medium for the selected method to become effective.

The duration of counselling will depend on various factors. It could be said that bereavement does not fit easily with short-term approaches such as solution-focused brief therapy and CBT because the central task is not to focus on solutions to problems. However, it may be enough to learn some strategies for coping with new realities.

Bereavement counselling may be sought at a time when the client is preparing for a transition to another stage in post-bereavement adjustment, and so may have fulfilled its purpose when, say, a bereaved father is re-established at work, or a bereaved mother is pregnant again. On the other hand, it could be precisely at this time that the newly pregnant woman experiences a *greater* need for counselling – particularly if the death was of a baby – so perhaps the real message here is not to make assumptions. Counselling in response to what may be regarded as complicated grief reactions is more likely to be long term, maybe lasting more than a year. In reality the number of sessions may depend on the regulation of the profession described above. Counselling from a private practitioner will offer more flexibility, but will depend on ability to pay.

For more on different aspects of bereavement counselling and when it is appropriate, *see Gift of Tears* by Lendrum and Syme (1992).

How is bereavement counselling different from other counselling?

Bereavement counsellors are sometimes referred to as a special breed. In fact, the title simply denotes a chosen area of specialism, and all counsellors will deal with bereavement to a lesser or greater degree. It could even be said that the issue of loss is central to all counselling. Having said that, there are some strategies that are associated with grief work, particularly to facilitate the expression of grief in situations where the mourner feels 'stuck'. Such strategies include the following:

➤ The construction of geneograms to identify patterns of loss and other affective factors in the family. This means of 'plotting' the family has proved to be one of the most useful tools in the author's toolbox, and is recommended as a routine opening to the counselling relationship. (*See* Appendix D for a sample diagram and guidelines for compiling a geneogram.)

➤ The use of photographs, videos and memorabilia as sensory triggers to access emotional memory.

➤ The use of the written word, both in the reading of literature and poetry, and through the client's own writings.

➤ The use of drawing and painting in free expression, which bypasses the need for words and helps to access feelings more directly.

➤ *In vivo* work, i.e. the revisiting of the scene of the death, the hospital where the death occurred, the grave, or other significant places. This may be done by the client alone, with others, or with the counsellor.

➤ The use of letters, tapes or 'empty chair' work, to help the client deal with 'unfinished business' – to express unspoken thoughts and feelings to the person who has died.

➤ Helping the client to devise and carry out personalised rituals to say goodbye or commemorate the life/death. This may be useful when the mourner has for some reason missed the funeral.

➤ Working with the whole family, perhaps in conjunction with another counsellor. This may be particularly appropriate regarding child loss, to avoid the false separation of issues and exclusion of some family members, usually siblings.

Some of these techniques are very powerful and should only be used when the counsellor has experienced them first-hand in the training setting, and can discuss their application in supervision.

Where should counselling take place?

The usual setting is a designated space in the counsellor's consulting rooms or the health practice, hospital or organisation where the counsellor works.

This affords privacy, freedom from interruption, standard conditions and safety for both parties. It denotes a special time and place for the client and the client's changing relationship with the dead child. Coming to the counsellor may also be seen as a test of commitment to engaging with painful feelings and difficult issues that arise. All these factors have contributed to the view that counselling in the client's home is second best, where the counselling may be subject to distractions such as pets, visitors and other family members.

On the other hand, home visits offer many bonuses, the client is seen in context, in terms of family and culture; the client may have more confidence in familiar surroundings, feel more in control of a new experience; and some might only engage in counselling on home ground. Above all, the home visit may indicate respect for the dead child in the place where he once lived and to the family holding his memory. In this regard office consultations are no substitute for home visits.

Certainly, counselling in the home requires more flexibility from the counsellor, as well as secure boundaries. Where there is a choice, the pros and cons would need to be considered as part of ongoing assessment and supervision.

Availability of counselling

The first consideration is whether there is someone already involved and acceptable to the bereaved person who can meet the criteria given above in terms of having awareness, training, time and supervision.

If so, it is important that the counselling is set up separately from other activities, and has clear time limits. If these conditions are not met, it may be difficult for both to cope with the painful feelings aroused. Professionals for whom counselling is a secondary role will arrange to see someone at a time set aside for addressing the bereavement issues. Referral through the GP will have set pathways from a central referral point after assessment of 'symptoms'.

In some parts of the UK there are bereavement centres or services with counsellors who have particular experience of working with grief. This was how Pam came to counselling:

> 'I lost my son 12 years ago. I thought I was managing OK but after a few years I was back and forth to the doctor with one thing and another – pains across my shoulders, down my back, stomach ache . . . He was very good: in the

end he said that either I went to a counsellor or he wouldn't be my GP any more! So I had no choice, though I didn't see it would do any good. In fact once I got there I realised how much I had been holding in and how much I needed to talk about my feelings. I grieved in a way I hadn't allowed myself to do before. I still need to talk about Simon from time to time. If I don't, the feelings come from nowhere and hit me in the back of the neck.'

Where a referral system operates within bereavement centres, it is important that the bereaved person is encouraged to self-refer, as it could be that a third party referral is more about the referrer's anxiety to help than the bereaved person's wish to be helped. Similarly, response to referrals should be directly with the bereaved, and thought given to how much information, if any, is shared with other professionals.

Every counsellor, whether self-appointed or working within an organisation, should be able to provide the enquirer with information about their code of ethics, training and ways of working.

Psychotherapy

The distinction between counselling and therapy is a fine one. In the USA the words 'therapy' and 'therapist' are more or less synonymous with 'counselling' and 'counsellor' in the UK. To add to the confusion, some counsellors in the UK describe themselves as psychotherapists on the grounds that they are doing the same work.

What, then, is the difference? As a generalisation, those who describe themselves as psychotherapists tend towards a more psychodynamic approach, which facilitates the resolution of underlying conflicts of separation, probably from childhood. The psychotherapist may then work actively with the transference of feelings that occur in the therapeutic relationship. Anyone with deep-seated personality problems would be better suited to this psychodynamic approach. The psychotherapist may use specialist techniques belonging to a particular school of therapy. At the same time, some trained counsellors will use the same assessment skills and range of techniques. The blurred edges between the two definitions of counselling and psychotherapy are reflected in the current plans for regulation, which allow registered practitioners to call themselves by either title.

PSYCHOLOGY

Further distinctions need to be made for those seeking specialist help.

Generally speaking, referrals to a psychologist focus on behavioural concerns. The behavioural approach may be indicated for someone whose bereavement has led to entrenched phobic reactions, such as the panic attacks associated with agoraphobia. While the training for clinical psychology is traditionally behavioural in origin, the psychologist is not restricted to this approach. Referrals are assessed individually and the appropriate therapy is offered. Where children are concerned, this may take the form of play therapy, or work with the whole family. When the help of a child psychologist is engaged for grieving siblings who show distressing and persistent behavioural changes, it is essential that such help is seen by the child as supportive. Otherwise there is the real danger that the child is scapegoated for the parents' or family's difficulties and will be labelled as a 'problem'.

PSYCHIATRY

Traditional psychiatric support is seen to be appropriate in the context of mental illness, and concentrates on drug treatments. Although many bereaved parents do, for a time, experience mental chaos and fear they are going mad, this is different from the long term separation from reality that accompanies psychotic illness. Also, the depression that normally accompanies bereavement – the suppressing of painful feelings – needs to be distinguished from depressive illness, which is physically dysfunctional and requires medical treatment.

However, in some hospitals and child guidance centres, psychiatrists who work alongside psychologists and social workers offer a more flexible response and make use of other therapeutic skills. This multidisciplinary approach is also commonly used for family therapy. This may be the desired option when the death of a child results in family dysfunction. It has obvious advantages when one member of the family – usually another child – is carrying responsibility for all the family's distress. The desired outcome of involving all or some of the family members is to help each one acknowledge feelings and be acknowledged – thus helping the family adjust to its loss. (*See* Chapter 2, page 42–3, for more on the systemic approach.)

Family therapy may be available through the local health services, social services and voluntary agencies such as Barnardo's and the Children's Society.

Finally, a word about the value of these different therapeutic approaches. It is hard to get away from the assumption that those practitioners who have had more specialised training and are better paid also offer 'better' services. However, the worth of any counselling or therapy depends on the *quality* of the attention given to the bereaved person or family.

The word therapist comes from the ancient Greek 'therapon', a servant who freely chose to devote his life to giving attention to others' needs. To make the same point in another way, as the anti-psychiatrist RD Laing said, 'Treatment is about how you treat people'. The core qualities of warmth, empathy and respect form the basis of any supportive relationship. Carol found just these qualities in her befriender:

> 'Jenny saw me through the worst time, really. For the first months after James died I couldn't go out, not even to the shops. I felt I couldn't face anyone. I rang a helpline one evening, and after that Jenny came to see me every week till I got my confidence back. She knew just what I was going through, because she'd been there too. And I remember thinking, she's survived, so maybe I will.'

GROUPS

Meeting together with others to form a group is a powerful experience.

This is particularly true for those who feel isolated by the shattering effects of losing a child. Common bonds are formed by that shared experience, which cuts across differences in age, social status, education and religion. It can be enormously reassuring and enabling to hear others express similar thoughts and feelings, and to know they face similar difficulties. It can provide a safe environment for dropping the public mask of normality and owning inner struggles with pain, anger, guilt and frustration. Negatives are balanced by positives, so that one member can feed off another's hope or optimism.

Lin's daughter Yvonne, aged 15, was killed in a road accident while on holiday abroad. These are her recollections about attending a parents' group:

> 'It saved my sanity. I felt very lonely, and I used to feel as if I was going mad, talking to Yvonne as if she was still in the house; but when I heard others say

similar things, I thought "Thank God, it happens to them too". I felt I could just be *me* there, whether in a happy mood or at rock bottom. I could laugh without feeling apologetic, and cry without feeling ashamed.'

Groups can also be extremely threatening for the same reason, that shared feelings are intensified. For some, particularly in the early days of bereavement, it is just too much to consider anyone else's pain but one's own. Timing and preparation are therefore important for anyone joining a group. The nature of the group will also affect the outcome. Does it have a therapeutic purpose, or is it focused on shared activities? Is it exclusive to parents, to adults, or to families? Are affected children to be offered a separate group? Some children's bereavement projects have discovered the benefit of running two separate groups for children and their parents/carers at the same time.

Self–help groups

The main focus of the self-help group is mutual support. The structure is usually informal and the agenda set by the members. It often provides a network of support outside the group meetings, leading to new friendships. Although there is freedom from the leadership of outside helpers, someone will need to take on a facilitator role in terms of liaison and organisation. One model for self-help groups for bereaved parents is provided by The Compassionate Friends, with local co-ordinators who act as contact points.

One advantage of self-selection is the potential for minority groups to meet together, such as parents who have been bereaved of a child through suicide or murder.

Led groups

Support groups set up by professional or voluntary workers offer the security of leadership, which helps to facilitate the work of the group. The formation of the group may be in response to request or perceived need. The role of the leader(s) may be a passive one, keeping time boundaries and facilitating introductions; or it may be more directive, with structured meetings around themes or tasks. In any case, the leader will act as a kind of container for the group, which makes it a very stressful role. The importance of planning, clear aims, ground rules and good support/supervision for the leaders cannot be overestimated, and these issues will be addressed in Chapter 9. Obviously a therapeutic group requires skilled leadership.

The advantage of led groups for the members is that they are released from responsibility for the group and feel safer to express difficult feelings. There will also be a degree of detachment in the leader, which enables her to orchestrate the group, so that everyone who wishes to speak has an opportunity to be heard.

Structure – open or closed?

An open group is one that has a fluctuating membership, open to all-comers with a free option whether and when to attend. This flexibility is welcome to those who feel the need for support at particular times, and may not wish to attend when they are feeling specially vulnerable or when they are enjoying a 'good patch'. If there is no consistent core of members, however, it can be difficult for newcomers to build trust in the group. The fact that newcomers are joining the group all the time also means that open groups go on from week to week or month to month, without any natural end. Newer members may welcome this, reassured by the presence of bereaved people who are further on in their journey; longer-term members may eventually find it less helpful to be constantly drawn back to the early days of grieving. On the other hand, an open group has the advantage of doing away with expectations about how anyone should be or behave according to the length of their bereavement.

A closed group is one that has a selected membership over a fixed period of time, and is likely to be more structured than an open group. A fixed term group is the preferred choice of most professionals who act as facilitators for several reasons:

➤ it is more manageable in terms of their own commitment
➤ it promotes trust and continuity for the members, who are therefore able to risk more of their true feelings
➤ it prevents dependence
➤ it confronts the harsh reality of moving on.

A closed group seems more appropriate for those who share common features in their bereavement, for example a group of parents who have lost a child from the same illness in the same hospital over the same period of time. It is perhaps less appropriate for those whose loss leaves little chance of adjustment, such as parents who have lost an older child for whom they have cared over many years.

There are obvious advantages to setting limits on the life of a group, whether that marks the end of the group or provides a natural break before reconvening.

SOCIAL ACTIVITIES

Shared activity can be a wonderful therapy in its own right. It is particularly attractive to those who have no time for counselling or groups but who welcome the chance to mix with others who share their special experience. Social events, physical activity, fundraising organisation and committee work all provide the opportunity for oblique support. Purposeful activity seems to be a natural coping mechanism for many men who are distrustful of emotion or see themselves in the stronger supportive role in the family.

Children are usually better disposed towards doing things than talking about feelings they are unsure about. In the early 1990s, Alder Centre expeditions to Northumberland to swim with Freddie the dolphin proved enormously popular and provided the opportunity for bereaved siblings to share experiences that had marked them out in another way. Planning and preparation brought them together socially, and the encounters with Freddie gave them a sense of being special as well as different. For one of those youngsters, the adventure also gave her the confidence to talk about the death of her sister for the first time. Their families came together to watch video recordings and share photographs.

As well as reducing isolation, social activities for adults can be fun too! Quiz nights, country walks and shared holidays bring people together to enjoy the good things of life. These are not only welcome diversions but also affirmations of one's place in the world and the right to take pleasure in it alongside the pain of grief. This was the comment of one mother after a week spent in the Lake District with other parents:

> 'I now know the meaning of holidays and what they are for, which since the death of my child, I had forgotten.'

Shared family holidays can provide the opportunity to enjoy an activity again which may have lost its meaning.

SUPPORT FOR CHILDREN

Various references have been made to the difficulties surrounding children's support needs. Parents who are overwhelmed by their own grief may find it hard to attend to the needs of their surviving children. Adults struggle to gain access to the understanding and feelings of children who have not developed the emotional language to express themselves. Children seek to protect their carers from distress as much as their carers try to shield them from the painful reality of death. As a result, children often become 'the forgotten mourners' when a sibling or friend dies. For those helpers who are aware of children's needs, the question remains of how to provide for them – particularly when dealing with very young children – which will avoid problems later on.

The most important factor that determines how children cope with loss is the attitude of the parents. Young children suffer most the *secondary* losses, such as lack of attention and the loss of security in an ordered world, when a sibling dies. If the parents are able to include their other children in their experience of loss, keeping them involved and informed, while at the same time maintaining a sense of safety and security in the family, then they will cope well. Parents are best placed to answer a child's questions and provide reassurance to counter their fears and concerns.

It follows, then, that the best way of supporting children is through the parents. First of all that means providing adequate support for the parents. Second, parents can be briefed as to how best to support their other children at the time of the bereavement. Remind parents that children will 'read' the emotions around them and overhear conversations, and will ask questions either directly or indirectly. The Foundation for the Study of Infant Deaths and cot death associations have highlighted the needs of siblings, of publishing leaflets and training befrienders to raise the issues with parents. The Compassionate Friends also publish helpful articles on the grief of sibling children and teenagers and how to help them understand death.

Advice to parents for the benefit of children

➤ If at all possible, keep the family together.
➤ Keep children informed about what is happening. Even very young children will sense distress and need to know its cause. It is better for children to hear unpleasant things from their parents than from strangers.

➤ Answer children's questions as honestly as you can.

➤ Reassure them that the death of their brother or sister was not their fault or responsibility.

➤ Do not be afraid of using the word 'death'. Children get confused and worried by phrases such as 'gone to sleep' or 'taken by Jesus'. Avoid fairy tales to explain death, and do not be afraid to admit that you do not know all the answers. The more openly your family can talk about death, the easier it is for the child to accept it.

➤ Allow your children to feel sad, angry and all the natural feelings of grief, although do not expect them to feel sad all the time.

➤ When young children include some aspect of the death in their play, this is normal and healthy. The same goes for telling strangers 'My little brother is dead'.

➤ Do not be afraid to show your own grief in front of your children. This will help them to grieve, and reassure them that you loved the child who died.

➤ Give constant reassurance that you love and care equally for these children too. Give them special times, and listen.

➤ Do ask for help if you feel unable to deal with your children during this time.

If parents are not able to be the primary carers for a while, or are emotionally incapable of giving this kind of attention, then many of the above tasks can be undertaken by a relative. The family may enrol the help of a member of the clergy, a teacher, a social worker or a health visitor to talk to a child or answer her questions. This should always be done in consultation with the parents, and if possible in their presence.

How far should a professional take the initiative in cases where the parents seem unaware of their child's needs? Such situations require great sensitivity in explaining to parents the cause for concern and gaining their co-operation. Working with the parents to win their trust brings the best chance of success.

In any case, talking to a child about death and allowing the expression of bereft feelings cannot be done in a vacuum. It needs to be done within the context of a trusting and caring relationship, with time for the child to talk and react.

See Chapter 6 for further guidance on talking with children and for information on behavioural reactions.

Innovative groupwork and projects for children

It has long been recognised that bereaved children have special needs, and that most children benefit from meeting with other bereaved siblings. This recognition has resulted in the development of groups for children where their needs can be addressed in the supportive setting of being with others who have had similar experiences. For some children this is therapeutic in itself. At the beginning of a group for bereaved siblings when group members were introducing themselves, I remember the relief shown on the face of a boy of 12 when he realised that another group member had also lost *two* siblings, as he had, and he no longer felt a freak.

After the reassurance of shared experience, the group offers ways of revisiting grief issues, understanding their losses and celebrating memories, of discovering ways of relating and having fun. Northamptonshire Social Services have developed a group work approach that has been echoed in many other parts of the country, offering youngsters the opportunity to socialise, work together and play together within a structure of activities planned by concerned and committed professionals. They certainly need to be committed, as this work is demanding and time consuming in terms of preparation, practicalities, skills and emotional resources.

Typically, the group will meet for eight to 10 weekly sessions with a structured programme that can be made flexible to the members' needs.

The experience of the Stockport Children's Bereavement *Kingfisher* Project provided an effective model for running such groups. In the 1990s, a multidisciplinary team was made up of professionals from a variety of backgrounds – child psychology, Macmillan nursing, social work, health visiting – who contributed group work skills and their different experiences of working with children. Referrals came from health, education and social services, regarding children and young people whose difficult bereavements had led to concerns about their moods and behaviour. Each child and family was assessed before inviting the child to join an age-appropriate group, and the parents/carers to join a support group running at the same time as the children's group. Weekly group supervision of all the group leaders monitored the development of the groups as well as providing support for such emotionally demanding work. Evaluation of the groups brought overwhelmingly positive reporting of the benefits gained by individual children and their families. As happens all too often with such projects, uncertain funding halted the development of the Stockport Project.

Liverpool Children's Project, funded by The Children's Society, followed a similar path of development, though working within more flexible frameworks. The age range of the children in any one group was wider, the membership more variable, and the length of the group more open-ended. The content focused more on social activities and being with other children, rather than activities directly addressing loss experiences.

Also in Liverpool, the Alder Centre established two-day residential therapeutic breaks for bereaved siblings. These breaks were facilitated by counsellors at the Centre together with professionals from within the Hospital Trust (play worker, social worker, psychologist etc). Each group had a maximum of 12 members aged between five and 12, who had been bereaved for six months or more. A variation of this pattern was for the group to meet for five weekly sessions and then to spend a day together, with family involvement in the first and last sessions.

Most people have heard of the Winston's Wish Project in Gloucestershire, which has led the field in this pioneering work with children. A range of services now includes individual work and social activities for children, advice and information for parents and support for schools, as well as the Camp Winston residential weekends for children and similar weekends for parents, which have featured on television documentaries. Although it can only deal with referrals within the county of Gloucestershire, Winston's Wish has inspired the development of grief support programmes all over the UK, and the Project offers help to others through training and consultancy work. The Project's leaflet includes these words:

> 'At Winston's Wish we believe all our services should be routinely available to every family. Most families need straightforward support, *not therapy*. It is our aim to ensure that all bereaved families can have the services they need when they feel the time is right.'

Throughout their work the emphasis is on supporting the child within and through the family system. Specifically, their aims include the encourage-ment of open communication in families and helping families to find ways of remembering the person who has died.

All the projects mentioned above in some way involve the child's parents. This is a welcome move forward from services that aim to support children in isolation from their parents and families. Such a separation is not only a false one, but it compounds any feelings of isolation that the child may already have experienced during and after the death of her sibling. These are the comments of one bereaved parent, based on the experience of her own surviving child and observations of the experience of siblings in other families:

> 'The trouble is – and I know the lack of resources is a problem – child loss is often dealt with as separate issues for parents and siblings, without realising that the two cannot be separated. Dealing with siblings in isolation replicates what happens at home, that is, they are often excluded and isolated by their parents, and counsellors who work with bereaved parents may sometimes miss the effects on remaining children and family dynamics. Losing a child affects every family member differently, which in itself alters family structures.'

References

Lendrum S, Syme G. *Gift of Tears*. London: Routledge; 1992.

Wolfelt A. Companioning vs treating: beyond the medical model of treatment, parts 1–3. *Forum Newsletter of Assoc of Death Educ in Counsel*. 1998; 24: 4–6.

Further reading

Herbert M. *Supporting Bereaved and Dying Children and Their Parents*. Leicester: The British Psychological Society; 1996.

Hill L, editor. *Caring for Dying Children and Their Families*. London: Chapman & Hall; 1994.

CHAPTER 8

Support for schools

'Grief should be the instructor of the wise;
sorrow is knowledge.'

Byron

HOW SCHOOLS ARE AFFECTED

After the family, the school community contains the people most affected by the death of a child – friends, playmates, fellow students, teachers, auxiliary staff. Parents and governors form part of the wider school community. Whether the death is anticipated or sudden, it may well be the first bereavement experience for the child's peers and for younger teachers too. Close attachments are formed between children and their teachers, particularly in the infant and junior school, so that the death of a child may be a personal as well as professional loss. Teachers have a highly developed sense of responsibility, and if the death occurs when they are in charge, they will be vulnerable to extreme stress. Dealing with death is not easy for teachers who are confined by a culture of being in control and having answers. When dealing with their own emotions, they rarely have their own space to retreat to, and are constantly paying attention to the demands of large numbers of children throughout the school day.

For the pupils, the closer they were to the child and the circumstances of the death, the more profound will be the consequences in terms of self-esteem, concentration and attainment levels. Follow-up studies on survivors of the *Jupiter* cruise ship sinking in 1988 showed significant effects on academic performance, after comparing end-of-year exam results before and after the incident for survivors and for non-cruise students (Dagwell, Tsui and Yule, 1993).

Two longer-term studies on the effects of the sinking of the *Jupiter* by Yule, *et al.* have been published in the *Journal of Child Psychology and Psychiatry* (Yule, Udwin and Murdoch, 1990; Bolton, *et al.*, 2000). They show that, following the accident, 52% of the affected teenagers developed symptoms of post-traumatic stress disorder, mostly within the first weeks. 15% still experienced these symptoms 5–7 years later. Overall, there was a three-fold increase in mental health problems, and the survivors developed depression and anxiety disorders to a far greater extent than control groups. Thus, what seemed to some like a frightening but minor disaster has been shown to have had major consequences.

The impact on the school as an organisation is often underestimated by outsiders, sometimes even by school managers themselves. Tragedy and trauma carry the potential both for bringing out the best in people and for magnifying any underlying difficulties. Most deaths of school-age children will be as the result of critical incidents, so it is worth looking at what happens to organisations under stress. The model pictured in Figure 8.1 is derived from the work of Carolyn Attneave in helping to deal with community crises in Canada over a 20-year period.

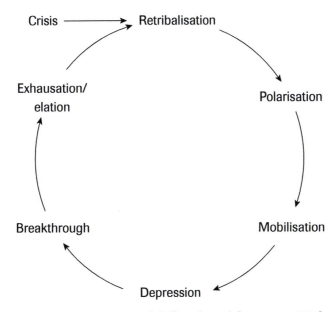

FIGURE 8.1 Response to crisis model (Speck and Attneave, 1973)

Observed phases help to understand and predict ways in which the school is likely to respond to crises:

1 *Retribalisation*
   This word describes the initial process of the community closing ranks, huddling together, wanting to keep out strangers etc. It is seen as a healthy early response to crisis and should be respected by outsiders seeking to help.

2 *Polarisation*
   A polarising of attitudes commonly occurs, for example between those who want to stop all normal activities and those who want to carry on as though nothing has happened. Healthy organisations can acknowledge and discuss these differences to prevent any destructive splitting. Help may be needed from outside to facilitate this.

3 *Mobilisation*
   If phase 2 has been negotiated, now people can begin positive action. Comfort is offered, connections made, feelings of loss and guilt are shared. Support from outside should concentrate on facilitating what others can do for themselves.

4 *Depression*
   This is the inevitable realisation that nothing will be the same again. A sense of despair spreads through the system as the absolute nature of the loss sinks in. The maintenance of support systems and monitoring of different needs are important.

5 *Breakthrough*
   Realisation of survival releases the potential to help others, while those who continue to feel helpless will remain in the depression phase. There may be a role for outside support to help different groups recognise their different stages and needs.

6 *Exhaustion/elation*
   Lack of sleep, exercise etc will catch up with people at this point and rest becomes necessary. Someone apart from the centre of things may need to say 'Go home now, you've done enough'. Another feature of this

phase may be pride and pleasure in having come through the crisis, and outsiders can help by recognising people's courage and coping.

Inner resources and outside help

Attneave's model gives some pointers as to when support from outside the immediate school community might be appropriate.

Schools are well used to dealing with crises, know their own systems, and develop their own coping strategies. The imposition of unbidden help from outside, however well meaning, will be counterproductive, as the result will be to disempower the school from using its natural resources. Also, strangers who come in to the school to talk to children about (the) death deny them the benefit of familiar and trusted adults to help restore their sense of security.

The experience of a Kidderminister school, after 12 of its children and a teacher were killed on the M40 in 1993, provided salutary lessons. Three teams of counsellors had arrived at the school on the first chaotic day after the accident, all of them unknown to the school – this simply added to the chaos. This experience highlighted the need for co-ordinated responses that first of all respect the school's natural resources – which in this case were

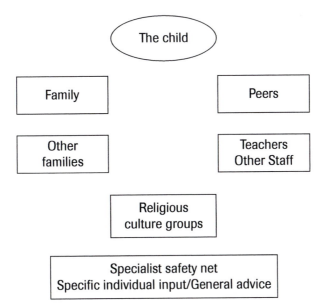

FIGURE 8.2 Bereavement support systems (O'Hara, Salford City Council training materials unpublished, originally used 1996)

rooted in the culture of the Roman Catholic church. The familiar local priest and parish helpers provided more effective support for this school than the teams of external counsellors.

The most efficient bereavement support systems are aptly illustrated in Figure 8.2.

O'Hara reminds us that those nearest to the child provide the most natural support. The 'specialists' from outside the community are better placed for supporting those who support the children, notably the teachers. Obviously, children need the love and comfort of parents and family when a child dies. The next most important adults are their teachers, who have a vital part to play as role models as well as educators. Usually they know instinctively what is best for the children, and will only need some reassurance that they can allow themselves to be open, honest and distressed in front of the children. When children are trusted with such openness they often surprise their teachers with their acceptance, generosity, imagination and resilience.

PLANNING AND PREPARATION

It is no surprise that schools deal better with a pupil's death if they are prepared. Although every situation is unique, and nothing can prevent feelings of shock and helplessness when the death occurs, there are common features that can be anticipated. Whether the death is expected or sudden, outcomes relate to three key areas: *communication, curriculum,* and *contingency plans.*

When the death is expected

Fortunately death from chronic illness such as childhood leukaemia or congenital disorder is now a comparatively rare event. Usually the family and school will keep in close contact as the disease progresses, and the class teacher is often the key link person. Communication is all-important, between family and school, between teachers and children. Conveying the seriousness of the situation as the child nears death, without conveying loss of hope, is a tricky task. However, preparation in some form facilitates the giving of the news when the child dies. Time and thought can be given beforehand as to how the children will be told, who attends the funeral, how feelings can be expressed and memories ritualised.

Good communication will depend partly on open and trusting relationships, and partly on how life and death issues are dealt with as part of the curriculum. As a generalisation it is probably true that there is now less of a taboo over discussing death with children, though how possible it is for children to explore death and dying will depend largely on how far teachers have tackled their own anxieties on the subject. In some schools 'death studies' are included in the PSHE curriculum, while related areas of study (including religious studies, biology, nature studies, and health and social care) all offer opportunities for developing understanding and vocabulary around death. Certainly it must help to deal with the death of a child if the school already has a language to speak in and reference points to use. (*See also* Chapter 6 on guidelines for talking with children.)

When the death is sudden

The death may be unexpected, as in the case of meningitis or an undiagnosed heart condition, or it may be as the result of a traumatic event – accident, murder, suicide, atrocity, disaster. It seems that man-made disasters such as Hungerford, Dunblane and the 7 July 2005 bombings in London are harder to come to terms with than natural disasters such as the Towyn floods. Again, public disasters carry more potential for shared experience and professional help, whereas private tragedies are more isolating and harder to deal with. There is plenty of research and literature now available to endorse the value of being as prepared as possible for the unexpected tragedy or critical incident. In 1993 all schools in the UK were issued with a free copy of *Wise Before the Event*, by William Yule and Anne Gold, funded by the Gulbenkian Foundation. This booklet spelt out clearly the case for making contingency plans that will lessen the impact on the school when a crisis occurs. Having argued the case for planning, to reduce the impact of physical and emotional effects of disaster, the authors offered strategies for schools to adapt and adopt as their own contingency plans. These guidelines have inspired many local authority initiatives to develop frameworks for the management and support of critical incidents and to encourage individual schools to set up their own protocols.

The work of Afra Ayalon in Israel, Atle Dyregrov in Norway, and Elizabeth Capewell in the UK has encouraged the shift from schools reacting to a crisis, to a prepared and proactive range of interventions. Otherwise the same principles apply as to expected deaths: children and their teachers benefit from good communication and awareness of death issues via the curriculum.

Specifically, what can schools do to prepare?

This process has been followed by many schools in recent years:

➤ set up a group of staff/governors to research the available literature, local guidelines and recent experience

➤ formulate an action plan (*see* below)

➤ establish a critical incident management team and identify key roles

➤ ensure that basic information, contact lists, communication systems and emergency procedures are in place and regularly updated

➤ carry out a simulation exercise to test out how a critical incident might unfold

➤ familiarise all staff and governors with action plans and procedures

➤ review the adequacy of curriculum coverage of death and loss issues

➤ identify training needs for staff.

The Local Authority (LA) has a crucially important role in supporting this process and responding to identified training needs. The relevant LA officer and other identified personnel should be on hand to offer practical support, and will probably act as key communication points within the school's action plan.

Trauma-related deaths of children will involve the emergency services, and the police will take control of certain procedures.

Action plans for managing critical incidents

As an example, West and East Cheshire LAs recommend the following action plan to its schools as a structure that can be readily adapted to most situations (Cheshire County Council 2007). Other LAs offer similar models, based on the *Wise Before the Event* booklet. This plan assumes that the school has a critical incident management team with identified roles.

Within hours:

➤ gather information about what has happened

➤ brief the critical incident management team, and allocate responsible adults to places where they are needed, e.g. hospital, child's home, administrative support

➤ use LA support network through designated contacts

➤ allocate space as an incident management room with an exclusive phone line or use of a mobile phone

➤ contact families whose children are involved, and make arrangements for informing other parents
➤ inform teaching and support staff
➤ inform the pupils
➤ be ready to deal with the media.

As soon as possible:
➤ prepare strategies for handling the reactions of people affected (*see* below)
➤ anticipate further information bulletins for parents not directly involved
➤ anticipate further media interest; liaise with the LA press officer or public relations department.

These pointers can act as a very useful checklist at a time when shock, panic and feelings of helplessness can threaten to overwhelm the most competent of school managers.

A question often faced in the immediate aftermath of a traumatic death is *'should the school be closed?'* There may, of course, be practical and safety factors to take into account. Psychologically, it is likely to be a mistake to assume that people – children or staff – are better off at home. Excepting the case of a school-based atrocity such as Dunblane, people need to be with others similarly affected after traumatic events to share their reactions, and people need the security of familiar faces, places and routines to help them through the dislocation of the first days.

The school is also a natural community meeting place for parents, many of whom will be drawn to the school for information and reassurance. Schools often find themselves unprepared for this, and surprised that the bereaved parents usually want to visit the school soon after the death. Anecdotally, this happened in one primary school the same day that the child died, much to the consternation of the headteacher, who felt inadequate to face distraught and possibly angry parents. In the event, the parents simply wanted to be where their child should have been that day, and to make contact with the other adults who had been such an integral part of their child's life. The headteacher and classteacher felt as comforted by the parents as the other way round.

PSYCHOLOGICAL SUPPORT: WHO DOES WHAT AND WHEN?

Two important guiding principles have already been established.

1 Schools cope better with the death of a pupil when they have established systems of communication. This applies to the ethos of the school, its ability to talk about emotional needs, as well as to protocols for conveying information.

2 A school's natural support resources need to be respected, especially with regard to the emotional needs of grieving children.

Having said that, there is a time and place for external supports. First, school staff who are providing support for children in their roles as closest trusted adults, will themselves need support. The concept of Winnicott's 'nursing triad' applies here, in that the primary carer needs to be 'held' to sustain the role, particularly when that caring role involves the containment of negative emotions.

Second, staff have their own grief to deal with, which may expose them to other personal griefs and anxieties, and some may feel the need for more support than can be offered by colleagues. Third, there will be incidents involving the death of a child when teachers and other school staff are so directly involved in the trauma as to be incapacitated themselves, either physically or emotionally.

The catch-all term for any kind of emotional or psychological support is 'counselling', as in media accounts which report that 'counselling will be available to the survivors' and 'counsellors are at hand at the site of the incident'. Local and national government members may also seek reassurance from school managers that *counsellors* are involved, as demonstrating that all is being done that is possible and that specialist help is being provided. The reality is that counselling is a specific kind of support not appropriate to the immediate situation. An analogy from the medical world might be to send for a physiotherapist when first aid is required! Sadly, some families after Lockerbie and Dunblane experienced inappropriate, untimely 'counselling' as intrusive.

Another expectation that has developed after major incidents is that a telephone helpline should be set up. The value of a helpline has been questioned, in that it may actually foster helplessness and anxiety in callers. Unless the helpline has a clearly defined remit, such as the provision of practical information following a meningitis outbreak, it may well prove to be a knee-jerk reaction to feelings of helplessness in those who want to help, or want to be seen as helping.

In order to clarify what kinds of psychological help are appropriate at different times, it will be useful first to consider the needs commonly experienced in reaction to the traumatic death of a child in a school community, and then to relate these needs to different levels of support.

Common reactions

Obviously reactions will vary according to the grieving individual's age and experience, the nature of the death and other circumstances, though it is possible to anticipate common emotional reactions. Not surprisingly, the most common reactions include *denial, distress, guilt, anger, helplessness*.

For those closely affected by a critical incident fatality, common reactions will include some of the classic post-traumatic stress symptoms associated with increased levels of arousal, re-experiencing the event, and avoidance of trigger stimuli. These can be simply understood as the stressful tension between the need to remember what has happened – in order to believe it and make sense of it – and the need to forget what has happened, because it is too painful or overwhelming. Normal reactions to these abnormal events commonly include *hyper-anxiety, irritability, sleep disturbance, flashbacks, detachment, lack of concentration, survivor guilt*.

The impact of a traumatic death on the school as an organisation can also be predicted (*see* pp 165–6). Existing strengths and vulnerabilities are likely to be magnified, and polarities may develop between different parts of the school community as it struggles to come to terms with what has happened.

Common needs

It follows from the above that common needs can be anticipated and certain actions taken to provide the best conditions for the school's recovery and to look after the mental health of its pupils and staff.

➤ Prompt, accurate and regular information about the incident is top priority. Anxiety and anger are fuelled by uncertainty and delay.

➤ As soon as possible, the school management needs to acknowledge what has happened and the sadness or horror of it, perhaps via year assemblies, class announcements, letters home.

➤ Staff and children need the opportunity to talk about what has happened, to ask questions, and to express their personal reactions.

This is most naturally done in familiar small groups, though it may also be appropriate to set aside a dedicated space in school where people can come and talk together about the dead child(ren) and find ways to express their thoughts and feelings in writing and drawing. Extra staff meetings give the opportunity to process reactions, monitor developments and work through different perspectives.

➤ There is a need for the school to connect with the dead child's family and wider community through informal contacts and formal rituals. Families usually welcome the active participation of the school in the funeral arrangements and their own involvement in school memorial services. In the longer term, anniversaries should be planned for and handled with sensitivity.

➤ When something dreadful has happened, there is a need for the security of familiar faces and surroundings and normal routines. Alongside the recognitions and rituals, the continuity of the school day and regular activities provide some measure of reassurance in a world suddenly made unsafe and unpredictable. Where staff are incapacitated, governors and parents can prove invaluable classroom assistants.

➤ Those providing front-line support, including administrative and auxiliary staff, need their own support. Relief cover should be anticipated for key staff who face additional stresses such as dealing with the media or anxious visitors. Senior managers, who usually cope very well with the immediate crisis, should be prepared for the time when their personal reactions catch up and need attention.

➤ Teachers and children who survived the fatal incident will need special support on their return to school. Discussion and planning will aid reintegration.

Siblings have their own special needs and present particular challenges to the school. Older children should be consulted as to how their peers and teachers can best help, and younger children given opportunities to express their feelings through drawing and play.

> 'Schools represent continuity for children in times of crisis. When a traumatic event directly strikes a school, it is important that the school continues as a supportive and stable part of the students' environment.' (Dyregrov, 1998)

LEVELS OF SUPPORT FOLLOWING CRITICAL INCIDENTS AFFECTING SCHOOLS

The following levels of support are suggested as another way of looking at who does what and when.

Level 1 'Someone there': The first hours

This is a mix of practical and emotional support at the time of the incident or in the immediate aftermath. The school head or other members of the senior management team may be in shock, and reactions may range from panic and helplessness to cool detachment. Appropriate support from outside the school means having someone to turn to for help in assessing the situation, working through the priorities and identifying available resources. Having someone at the end of the phone may be sufficient, though in many cases the physical presence of someone going out to the school – perhaps at the end of the day – is very reassuring.

Level 2 'A listening ear': The first days

Soon after the event there is a need for most people to talk – about what has just happened, about their immediate reactions and concerns. Support requirements at this stage may include reassurance, information, guidance or advice, but is essentially the ability to listen, accept and understand – basic listening skills. Practical support for the school head may be appreciated in the form of letter templates, script examples for telling children bad news, useful leaflets to send to parents etc. Requests to outsiders to become directly involved with children at this stage should be resisted, in favour of helping heads and staff to re-engage with their own resources.

Level 3 'Structured Group Debriefing': The first weeks

Those people directly affected by the incident may benefit from the provision of a structured meeting to process what has happened and to identify helpful resources. This form of group debriefing was developed by Mitchell in the US and by Dyregrov in Europe, and as part of an integrated package of care it has been valued as a supportive and educational strategy. Group debriefing includes 'acknowledgement of the psychological impact of traumatic incidents . . . reassurance about immediate distress, and information about the likely course of symptoms' as part of the 'general, practical and social support and guidance to anyone following a traumatic incident' recommended in Department of Health NICE guidelines. This structured group support is facilitated by trained personnel and follows established protocol regarding selection, conditions, process and timing (not too soon after the event). Single session debriefing of individuals is **not** to be recommended, however.

(For more information on debriefing and post-traumatic stress disorder (PTSD), refer to NICE guideline 26, NO849, sections 7.1–7.5.)

Level 4 'Counselling': The first months

Those whose post-traumatic stress reactions persist and cause difficulties and which hinder the return to normal functioning will need individual therapeutic intervention. GPs normally take responsibility for the assessment and coordination of care of PTSD sufferers and will refer on to specialist services within the NHS. Recommended therapeutic approaches include CBT and Eye Movement Desensitisation and Reprocessing or EMDR.

Others who continue to be affected but do not qualify for a medical diagnosis may also benefit from counselling and may seek appropriately qualified practitioners via Occupational Health (for staff), voluntary organisations or privately.

Advice and guidance

The school will benefit from having access to advice and guidance throughout their experience of the death of a pupil. There is an ongoing process of monitoring reactions and assessing support needs, and even the most self-sufficient school community will usefully refer to outside resources for reassurance and support.

At a stressful time, school managers are likely to turn to someone who is already known to the school, so it may be worth the effort to make contact with any specialist resources for advice and guidance *before* they are needed. They may have useful information to offer on how other schools have managed similar situations; on which children will be particularly vulnerable; on useful reading materials and references. Does the LA have an adviser with responsibility for such advice and guidance? For independent and private schools, is there access to an external consultant?

In certain situations and at certain times, consultation will appropriately lead to the direct intervention of external support; but for the most part the consultant's job is to empower teachers and school managers in using their own skills and resources.

What of those schools whose managers adopt the 'stiff upper lip' to emotional distress and deny the impact on the school, themselves or others? There is no doubt that the headteacher's attitude is a crucial factor, and s/he acts as a role model for staff and children. Senior managers promote the ethos of the school and its value system. It is their responsibility to assess the needs of staff and pupils in the light of what is now known about the impact of life-threatening events and sudden death. In this task they are accountable to parents, governors and to the wider community.

If the school is intolerant of emotional need, the following myths may operate:

➤ 'Infants don't understand about death, are not affected, don't need to be told.'
➤ 'The child who died didn't go to our school, so there's no need to mention it.'
➤ 'The children will lose confidence in their teachers if they see them upset.'
➤ 'We have a wonderful pastoral system, so we don't need any help.'
➤ 'The children don't seem to be upset, so they must be all right.'
➤ 'Encouraging the expression of feelings will lead to mass hysteria.'

Challenging such myths needs to take place *before* the death of a child, at a time when these defences are not so strong. Assessment and review of the school's contingency plans and curriculum provision are good places to start. These processes can be initiated by anyone from a range of interested people, including staff, parents, governors, advisers and inspectors.

AFTER A SUICIDE (*see also* Chapter 6, Guidelines for talking with children)

Suicide is difficult to contemplate and talk about, and all the more so when it is a young person who has apparently chosen to end his own life. How can a young person, with his whole life ahead of him, make a conscious choice to die? The word suicide carries the notion of intent, and therefore it is unwise to use it before the coroner's verdict. In the absence of a written statement, it may never be possible to know whether the death resulted from a deliberate decision, or was the accidental outcome of a bizarre experiment. On the other hand, where it is clear from the facts that the young person died by his own hand, it is also unwise to protect others from the truth by describing the death simply as 'sudden' or 'tragic'.

This situation is a minefield for school managers faced with informing the school community, supporting the parents, handling the immediate publicity, and then coping with the questions and soul-searching that inevitably follow. From the start, the authority's press officer needs to be involved, and consultative support needs to be available.

Of course the young person's immediate peers and teachers will be greatly affected and may need intense support. But all the staff will be hit hard, and the ripples of shock and disbelief will continue through the governors, other parents, and the community at large. Everyone will be asking, of themselves and of others: Why? What signs did we miss? Could we have done more? Could it have been prevented?

Knowing that these are natural reactions can provide some helpful guidance as to what reassurance is needed for the school community. It helps to know that feelings of *guilt* (should I have picked up on something?); *rejection* (why didn't he talk to us?); and *despair* (the world is unsafe now, so could I do this too?) are commonly experienced.

Added to this, suicidal thoughts are quite common in adolescence anyway, as part of the normal developmental process, along with existential issues in general and trying to understand death and the meaning of life. It is really important to remember that young people bereaved through suicide will be more vulnerable to suicidal feelings of their own. Acknowledging this explicitly helps to normalise such feelings, whereas allowing the stigma of suicide to forbid talking about it can only magnify those fears.

The following extract is taken from a collection of experiences of people bereaved through suicide (*A Special Scar* by Alison Wertheimer). It is written by a young adult but is relevant to any age.

> 'Although I had never in my life contemplated suicide, one of my biggest fears after Ros's death was that I'd kill myself too. Only a few weeks after Ros died a colleague at work also hanged himself. That made things even worse. The world began to feel very unsafe. Two people in two months? I remember lying in bed after John's suicide looking at the curtain rail and thinking it would be quite easy to copy them . . . These feelings have almost completely disappeared now but at the time I kept them to myself, and there was no one to tell me that this is a common reaction to suicide.'

Here it is important to point out that reassurance about the 'normality' of suicidal thoughts or suicidal fears only carries the risk of normalising suicidal behaviour when the realisation of those thoughts becomes the only way out of life's difficulties. Unfortunately the Internet sites which encourage the sharing of suicidal thoughts in an irresponsible way may also serve to facilitate suicidal behaviours.

So what can schools do to minimise the risks of suicidal behaviours? Many of the variable risks relate to family circumstances, cognitive style and personality, and/or psychiatric disorders. The marked susceptibility to stress that follows makes it hard to cope with negative life events. Such events, which may then trigger attempts or suicide, include the break-up of relationships, a family disturbance, a failure in performance, bullying and victimisation. Although many of these factors belong outside of school life, it is usually – though not always – easy to identify those young people who are in serious distress through their behaviour in school. Knowing how to respond to distressed and suicidal students is much more difficult. While many school staff members have the necessary skills and resilience to treat such students with sensitivity, some may resist a pastoral role or fear facing their own psychological problems. The task of managing individuals at risk is best shared with support professionals and community mental health services.

The ethos of a healthy school is already committed to fostering positive self-esteem in students and to promoting their emotional development. Such a positive mental health approach is probably the most important aspect of suicide prevention. As well as promoting emotional expression and communication skills, schools can create a safe environment free of intolerance to help prevent bullying, and they can provide information about care services, making contact details of crisis and emergency helplines accessible.

Papyrus is a national UK charity that provides resources and support for parents and professionals, including teachers, dealing with young suicides.

Finally, the reader is reminded of the necessity to have emergency plans on how to inform staff, fellow pupils and parents when suicide has been committed or attempted.

Chapter summary of key points
- Don't underestimate the impact of a child's death on the school.
- Healing comes from within, supported by outsiders.
- Planning and preparation pay dividends.

- Reactions and support needs can be anticipated, and then matched with appropriate resources.
- Information and communication are paramount.
- People need permission to talk and cry.
- Rituals and normality restore security.

References

Bolton D, O'Ryan D, Udwin O, Boyle S, Yule W. The long-term effects of a disaster experienced in adolescence: II: general psychopathology. *J Child Psychol Psychiatry.* 2000; **41**: 513–23.

Dagwell K, Tsui E, Yule W. *Effects of a Disaster on Children's Attainment.* Unpublished.

Dyregrov A. Psychological debriefing – an effective method? *Traumatology.* 1998; **4**: 6–15.

Hindmarch C. Counsellors will be on hand. *CPJ.* 2001; **12**(9): 9–11.

O'Hara DM, Taylor R, Simpson K. Critical incident stress debriefing: bereavement support in schools – Developing a role for an LA educational psychology service. *Educ Psychol Pract.* 1994; **10**(1): 27–34.

Speck RV, Attneave CL. *Family Networks*, New York: Pantheon Books; 1973.

Wertheimer A. *A Special Scar: the experiences of people bereaved through suicide.* London: Routledge; 1991.

Cheshire County Council. *Managing the Response to Critical Incidents in Schools.* Chester: CCC; 2007. (Now separated into Cheshire East Council and Cheshire West and Chester.)

Yule W, Gold A. *Wise Before the Event.* London: Calouste Gulbenkian Foundation; 1993.

Yule W, Udwin O, Murdoch K. The 'Jupiter' sinking: effects on children's fears, depression and anxiety. *J Child Psychol Psychiatry.* 1990; **31**(7): 1051–61.

Further reading

Ayalon O, Flasher A. *Chain Reaction.* London: Jessica Kingsley; 1993.

Capewell E. Responding to children in trauma: a systems approach for schools. *Bereavement Care.* 1994; **13**(1): 2–7.

Dyregrov A. *Grief in Children.* London: Jessica Kingsley; 1994.

Job N, Frances G. *Childhood Bereavement: developing the curriculum and pastoral support.* London: National Children's Bureau; 2004.

Stuart J. The eyes have it – EMDR therapy. *The Independent*, 8 January 2003.

Teachernet. *Health and Safety.* Website developed by the Department for Children, Schools and Families, with lesson plans and PSHE resources. Available at www.teachernet.gov.uk/healthandsafety (accessed 28 June 2009).

CHAPTER 9

Support services

'The death of a child is not something to be joked about, or laughed at. It is an event from which a parent does not recover: life is never quite the same again, nor should be, for now it incorporates an unnatural event. We do not expect to outlive our children, nor do we want to. On the other hand, life must go on, if only for the sake of those who are left, and, what is more, it is our duty to learn to enjoy it again.

For what do we regret for those untimely dead, but the opportunity to live with enjoyment? If we are to give proper meaning and honour to their death, and our grief, we must enjoy the life we, and not they, are privileged to have, and live thereafter properly and well, without wranglings or rancour.'

Fay Weldon, *The Hearts and Lives of Men*

As the special needs of bereaved families and communities become better recognised, various initiatives are developed to provide support. Some thrive while others prove short-lived, and the difference between the two is often put down to chance. It will be proposed here that the success of any support service will depend first on meeting certain core conditions, and second on good planning and preparation. These will be applied to the setting up of a support group, but could equally well be applied to starting a helpline or befriending service. Finally, the way forward to improved bereavement care will focus on the need for co-ordinated services, better information and proactive support.

CORE CONDITIONS

Some basic principles apply to the establishment of any support service, whether it be a group, befriending, counselling or a multipurpose centre.

Identifying the need

This means consulting those who are perceived as needing support at the time. One difficulty is that people do not always know what they want in their distress, or whether the support being offered will suit them. In this case the helper can draw on the past experience of families and consult other professionals. Another possible factor is that well-meaning carers may be more concerned about 'doing something to help' than responding to actual need. Indeed, an assessment of support needs may indicate a separate agenda for the professional or volunteer, which will have to be recognised and accommodated.

Assessment also involves identifying existing means of support, to ensure that services are not duplicated.

Sufficiency of resources

Too often, bereavement support initiatives fizzle out for want of adequate resources. Perhaps after a first flush of enthusiasm, just a few volunteers are left to cope with too many demands. Sometimes an initiative will depend on the commitment of one dedicated individual, whose bereavement work is not recognised as part of the job: when that person moves on, the project collapses. Sufficiency of resources relates to people, time, space and money. Although the setting up of any new service requires an act of faith, it is irresponsible to do so without reasonable confidence that the service can be sustained over a period of time, especially when working with loss and grief.

Support systems

Care for the carers is essential in such an emotionally demanding area of work. Management and administrative structures are necessary to any support system, however informal.

Key questions need to be addressed at the research and planning stage relating to the type and scope of the proposed service.

➤ At whom is the service aimed?
➤ What does the service aim to achieve?
➤ What are the geographical boundaries?

➤ What is already being done?
➤ What is the preferred setting?
➤ Who will deliver the service?
➤ What are the criteria for taking referrals?
➤ Who will manage and supervise the work?

At all stages it is important to work co-operatively with those with common interests and seek their support. Bereavement projects, by nature of the subject, tend to attract defensive attitudes! Canvassing for a broad base of support also ensures that your plans are in line with progressive thinking and good practice in other areas.

STARTING A SUPPORT GROUP

The guidelines suggested here assume that professional or voluntary workers are responding to perceived needs of bereaved family members, which may be met by offering a group experience. For the sake of convenience I shall refer to the potential group participants as parents, although of course they may be grandparents or siblings. The process will be the same, except that a sibling group will need parental agreement, and its leaders will require some understanding of children's perceptions.

Identifying the need

The impetus to start a group tends to fall into one of three categories:
1 in response to requests from parents to meet other parents for mutual support
2 in anticipation of griefwork, which can be facilitated in a therapeutic setting
3 as an economical way of coping with limited resources to offer individual help.

Being clear about the purpose will affect the direction you take and determine the appropriate type of group (*see* Chapter 7 for an outline of different group types). Whatever the impetus, it is important not to be pressured into starting a group before adequate preparation. This may be frustrating for potential participants, who will welcome regular communication during the planning stages.

The consultation process includes an audit of what is happening elsewhere to avoid duplicating resources, and making links with other colleagues, agencies and disciplines to ensure a broad base of support for the venture. Management may require data to back up any application for time or other resources and to clarify issues such as confidentiality.

Calling a meeting

An open meeting of all interested parties needs a clear agenda, someone to take a chairing role and someone to take names and notes. If likely attenders of the group are not present, their views should be represented.

The primary purpose of this first meeting is to take an audit of concerns, current practice, interests and resources.

➤ It is helpful to begin with introductions by name, role, agency representation and reason for attending. Some may see this initiative as a means of getting recognition for the work they already do for bereaved families or to gain understanding of their own support needs: it is important that these concerns are acknowledged by the Chair so that they can be openly identified and separated from the parents' needs.

➤ The purpose of the group, in the kind of general terms that can be summarised in one sentence, should then be agreed.

➤ The type and status of group required can then be discussed, along with the implications for resources. It may not be possible to reach a consensus at this stage.

➤ Another audit follows of the kind of help and commitment attenders are willing and able to give.

➤ A *small* working party can now take the findings forward to the next planning stage. There tends to be a high level of enthusiasm at this first meeting, so beware the 'hands up to volunteer' approach! Some means of communicating progress needs to be agreed, and dates set if the working party is to report back to another general meeting.

Planning

The planning tasks cover objectives, method, structure and programme, and a number of meetings may be needed.

➤ *Objectives*: these spell out the aim and purpose in specific terms. What will the group need to achieve its purpose? What conditions need to be met?

➤ *Method*: what kind of group (open or closed, self-help or led, spontaneous or planned) will be most appropriate? What size, composition and setting will help to meet the objectives?

➤ *Structure*: this provides boundaries for the group and moves on to practicalities. These will include:
  ➣ setting dates for starting (and finishing)
  ➣ deciding the venue
  ➣ agreeing the personnel to facilitate the group
  ➣ guidelines for access, referral and selection
  ➣ publicity
  ➣ arranging support and supervision for leaders
  ➣ setting dates for evaluation.
➤ *Programme*: the facilitators/leaders of the group will need to be involved, if not already part of the working party, to plan timing, format and – if appropriate – the content of group meetings. If canvassing for participants, a rough guide to uptake is that one in three will respond. Parents who wish to attend the group should be visited beforehand if possible.

Delivery

Thought needs to be given to the preparation of the room, who will welcome the group members, how the group will start and how it will end. Finishing group meetings can be very difficult, but it is important to draw the session to a close, gently but firmly, at the time stated. Groups that go on till midnight are exhausting for all concerned. Parents who are overwhelmed by exposure to never-ending pain are likely to drop out. It helps if the facilitator signals the end of the session some minutes beforehand, and at the finish time physically leaves the room or puts the kettle on.

It is essential for those in charge of the meeting, whether called hosts, leaders or facilitators, to debrief their feelings and reactions before going home and ensure that time for this is built in.

Evaluation

Groups do not always turn out as expected, even after meticulous planning! Evaluation is part of the group process, and may lead to amendments as the group goes on. At another level, the facilitators' supervisor will help them to evaluate their contribution, celebrating achievements as well as learning from mistakes. Managers and funding bodies may also require evaluative reports. When the group is time-limited, evaluation may lead to the implementation of necessary changes if another group is proposed. Open-ended groups benefit from a break of some kind, perhaps over the summer, which provides a natural time for taking stock.

A CO-ORDINATED APPROACH

A co-ordinated approach may be understood as one which incorporates the provision of different services, or as one which enables different service providers to work co-operatively.

Various attempts have been made to provide a range of support services under one umbrella that are flexible to different needs. The Alder Centre in Liverpool modelled one such approach, followed by the Laura Centre in Leicester, both founded *to support* **anyone** *affected by the death of a child*.

The Alder Centre has a dual remit of care and education. Its relationship with Alder Hey Hospital means that it can coordinate a continuum of care from the time leading to the child's death, through the time of the death, until long after the bereavement. It is equally available to families and carers when a child has died in the community. The Centre caters for group as well as individual bereavement support, for befriending as well as counselling. It accommodates the needs of bereaved parents to keep in touch through a physical place where they can be with the memory of their dead children in a special way. Therapeutic breaks are organised for families and for siblings. This psycho-social approach to bereavement care forms a circular pathway back into the community.

The Centre also provides a resource for both the training and support needs of professionals who work with bereaved families. For example, regular contributions are made to medical student training programmes at the Alder Hey NHS Trust, and Family Liaison police officers who deal with road fatalities, to help them develop the sensitivity and skills needed to work with families following the death of a child.

The role of bereaved parents has been instrumental to the development of the Alder Centre from its inception in 1989. Initially, they guided policy and practice to make the services relevant to their needs. While professional staff offered detachment, particular skills and expertise, the voluntary involvement of parents provided authenticity. Parent participation was experienced as therapeutic, whether as conference speaker or tea-maker. Helping others gave more purpose to the lives they were rebuilding.

'Dot is one of the parents who worked tirelessly for the Centre from the planning stage in a number of different roles at various times. As her 13-year-old daughter was approaching death, Dot asked Christine, "What do you want me to do?". Christine's answer was, "Help someone else." In the voluntary tasks she has undertaken – answering the helpline, befriending, fundraising, talking to visitors – Dot felt that Christine was working alongside her. (*See* Chapter 10 for more on Dot's story.)

Jo, Eunice and Bernie are typical of volunteer parents whose work at the Centre has fed into their own personal growth and career development. All three have become qualified counsellors. Since her son Liam's death, Bernie has also graduated in Childhood Studies, which included a dissertation on sibling grief for which she gained an 80% rating. "I was really thrilled to get this result but also sad because the subject matter depended on the fact that my son, and the children of my friends who participated in the research, had died. I didn't want an honours degree in losing a child".'

The needs of parents at different times as either users or providers of services, or both at the same time, may be difficult to accommodate. As some parents find new ways of relocating their grief, a natural development may well be to move away from their resource base, while others need to maintain the same relationship to core services and contacts for many years. Perhaps this tension reflects the variety of ways in which parents forge 'continuing bonds' with children beyond death (*see* Chapter 2, pp 37–8). In spite of these difficulties, the benefits of bereaved parents and professional helpers working co-operatively are enormous and well worth striving for. The Centre was founded on the principle that both can learn from each other and give to each other. Training offers the ideal forum for this two-way process: staff can train parents as telephone helpline befrienders; while the experience of parents can provide valuable input to training programmes for professionals.

This strong and comprehensive partnership of lay volunteers and professionals remains unique within the NHS.

The way forward
How can support services for those affected by the death of a child be improved? Specifically, the trend appears to be towards more inclusive family work, rather than splitting off mothers, fathers and siblings artificially. This approach makes a lot of sense but requires flexible and well-staffed

resources. The support resources available to a bereaved family, and to their carers, all too often seem to be a random affair, depending on where people live. Comprehensive systems such as the Alder Centre are probably only practicable in association with a children's hospital or hospice. Those living in a sparsely populated rural area have a slim chance of finding a support group within easy travelling distance. On the other hand, everyone has access to primary healthcare services and, through them, should have access to regional and national services.

Health visitors are well placed to provide such frontline support to families. A study conducted by Ann Dent in 1996 showed that families are particularly vulnerable to isolation when the death of a child is sudden and unexpected (Dent, 1996). Following this study, interventions were devised to empower health visitors in their support of 167 suddenly bereaved families over a two-year period in the South and West of England. At the end of this time a follow-up study showed significant improvement in the way families felt supported. It is interesting to note that these families felt better supported informally, via friends and neighbours, as well as formally, through the help of professionals such as the health visitor.

It is also important to recognise the value of the role that education can play in supporting bereaved families. In our Western society, which thankfully sees few child deaths and does not deal well with death generally, young parents may be totally unprepared for their grief reactions. Few will have experienced previous bereavements or had the opportunity to observe others' grief. Arguably, bereavement support, which includes an educative element to prepare them and to normalise even the most extreme of their reactions, will help to prevent complicated grief responses that become disabling and in need of crisis intervention at a later stage.

There is a clear case for auditing and co-ordinating bereavement support services, working towards a standard provision of care. The National Association of Bereavement Services did much to address this need. More recently, the Childhood Bereavement Network (CBN) has drawn up a databank of organisations and individuals providing bereavement services for children, has set up regional groups to network and develop local services, and has produced a comprehensive range of educative resources for schools (see Appendix C). The CBN operates under the umbrella of the Childhood Bereavement Project, a multi-agency initiative funded by the Diana, Princess of Wales Memorial Fund and hosted by the National Children's Bureau.

How proactive should bereavement care services be? The usual expectation of a bereavement support agency is that bereaved parents themselves make contact, or that a third party referral is received by a concerned professional, friend or relative. Yet it is well known that the bereavement experience leaves some parents paralysed by shock, floating in a limbo of grief that renders them incapable of asking for help. Agoraphobic responses are common and members of minority groups are naturally reluctant to use mainstream services. All these factors beg the question whether support services should initiate contact, or whether this would amount to an invasion of privacy.

The Kinder–Mourn Project in North Carolina, USA, is a community support agency modelled on The Compassionate Friends, who will *initiate* contact with bereaved parents brought to their attention by anyone concerned for their welfare. Home visits as early as the day of the funeral point the way towards informal parent support groups led by trained facilitators. In our more conservative British society, such proactive outreach is a less familiar concept; but arguably there is much to be achieved by support agencies reaching out to those who are unable to ask for help themselves. It is hoped that this book will give confidence to professionals to co-ordinate and advertise existing resources, and to experiment with more proactive means of support.

The guidelines offered here aim to encourage the faint-hearted as well as the visionary, and to affirm the good practice of those already engaged in providing bereavement services. Support is a two-way process. Families want information, choices and understanding. Professional carers need assurance that they *can* and *do* help by providing information and choices, and above all by being available to accompany the family on their journey through grief.

Reference

Dent A. A study of bereavement care after a sudden and unexpected death. *Arch Dis Child*. 1996; 74(6): 522–6.

CHAPTER 10

Hope, meaning and resilience

'When it is dark enough, you can see the stars.'

Charles A Beard

THE RIPPLING EFFECT

There is one resource that is easily overlooked, and this is the source of strength that can come from the bereaved parent's continuing relationship with the child after death. This does not require a belief in the spirit world or an afterlife, but a recognition that every life, however short or limited, leaves its mark. There are ways in which the 'continuing bonds' (*see* Chapter 2, pp 37–8) provide inspiration and help to build resilience.

In a recent publication, the existentialist psychotherapist Irvin Yalom has explored the concept of *rippling*, referring to the fact that everyone creates circles of influence which affect others who survive them.

> 'That is, the effect we have on other people is in turn passed on to others, much as the ripples in a pond go on and on until they're no longer visible but continuing at a nano level. The idea that we can leave something of ourselves, even beyond our knowing, offers a potent answer to those who claim that meaninglessness inevitably flows from one's finiteness and transiency.' (Yalom, *Staring at the Sun*, 2000, p. 83)

Following Yalom's notion of this rippling effect, every child's life has an impact, first on its parents and immediate circle, and through them to a wider community. This is more readily observable when the child who has died has made an obvious contribution, through their admirable qualities, good looks, or worthy achievements. Less obvious, after the ordinary miracle of birth itself, is the love and joy generated by a child's trust, affection, curiosity, and potential. Of course every child is special to its parents, but if his or her existence in any way enriched the lives of the parents, then that specialness lives on, in and through others. Even young babies have made some contribution. Continuing bonds can bring continuing gifts.

The reader is referred back to Chapter 2, p 39, where the concept of positive psychology is explained. It is concerned with the positive human qualities that underpin optimum functioning. Greater understanding has emerged of psychological resilience, and how it is that some people can incorporate life's adversities and adapt to them successfully. Such people are able to resist the kind of helplessness which comes from believing that bad things always happen to them and blame themselves when they do. There will be individual and social circumstances that affect this ability to resist helplessness. Machin (2007) identifies three common elements that characterise resilience:

1 *personal resourcefulness* – involving qualities of flexibility, courage and perseverance
2 *a positive life perspective* – which includes optimism, hope, a capacity to make sense of experience and motivation in setting goals
3 *social embeddedness* – in which support is available and there is the personal capacity to access it.

The psychoanalyst Cyrulnik is well known in his native France for the work he has done on childhood trauma and on helping to heal the wounds left on France by the Second World War. His own parents died in Auschwitz. He also believes that resilience results from a process that requires the right conditions. He argues that it is not simply a character trait, and that people are not born more or less resilient than others. His book on resilience has now been published in English (Cyrulnik, 2009). In an interview for the Family section of the *Guardian* newspaper, he is quoted as saying:

> 'Resilience is a mesh, not a substance. We are forced to knit ourselves, using the people and things we meet in our emotional and social environments. When it is all over and we can look back at our lives from heaven, we say to ourselves: "The things I've been through. I've come one hell of a long way. It wasn't always an easy journey". (*Guardian*, 18 April 2009)

Those who develop resilience are shown to have the capacity to grow through adversity in the following ways, according to Joseph and Linley:

'First, people often report that their relationships are enhanced in some way, for example, that they now value their friends and family more, and feel an increased compassion and altruism towards others. Second, survivors change their views of themselves in some way, for example, that they have a greater sense of personal resiliency, wisdom and strength, perhaps coupled with a greater acceptance of their vulnerabilities and limitations. Third, there are often reports of changes in life philosophy, for example, survivors report finding a fresh appreciation for each new day, and renegotiating what really matters to them in the full realisation that life is finite . . .

There is a shift from the self-perception as a victim to that of survivor. However, trauma survivors embrace this positive approach to life within a context of tragic hopefulness. They know firsthand the ups and downs, and the limits of human life. This awareness guides them to live their lives in a way that is truly and positively authentic, interpreting their trauma as a valued learning opportunity and giving back to others through the benefit of their experience.' (Joseph and Linley, 2006, p. 124)

Having survived the cruellest of blows, bereaved parents can discover hidden strengths and learn to foster unknown talents. Alongside their enduring grief, parents can derive supportive comfort from photographs, memorabilia, visits from the child's friends, anniversaries. They may use their own experience to offer understanding and support to those more recently bereaved who are struggling to find hope and meaning in their lives. Some may choose to give time and energy to existing support services, perhaps those from which they have benefited in the rawness of their grief, as volunteer befrienders or fundraisers. They may be inspired to establish new services where there is a gap in provision. From the manner of their child's death, they may develop a determination that the future is somehow better, that their child has not died in vain. Anger at the injustice of it all can provide the energy and driving force behind fundraising activities, and campaigns to improve services or challenge perceptions. Finding some way of honouring the life and memory of the child can help build the resilience needed to cope with the aching hole that has been left.

In all these different ways bereaved parents may seek to use their child's legacy positively to make the world a better place. The same motivation may apply to professionals who have devoted their working lives to helping others because they have been touched by the life and death of a child.

The stories which follow are based on interviews with parents who have lost children in very different circumstances. What they have in common is a shared hope for a better future and a determination to give meaning to their child's life. The experience of grief can breed despair and bitterness; equally it can develop personal qualities that improve one's own and others' lives. And, of course, it can move between these two polarities.

The message of these stories is: that which does not kill you *can* make you stronger. Resilience is a gentler word than strength. It implies the ability to survive one storm, the better to withstand another. The use of this word also reflects the acknowledgement that positives can come from negatives and that all life experiences carry the potential for learning and growth.

SOME PARENTS' STORIES

DOT AND CHRISTINE

Dot and Bob were looking forward to having a large family. After seven years and three miscarriages they were thrilled when Christine was born in 1971. Repeated chest infections led to a diagnosis of cystic fibrosis, when Christine was 18 months old. They had never heard of cystic fibrosis. At the end of their first consultation they were stunned to hear the paediatrician say, 'Of course, a cystic fibrosis child never lives into adulthood'. They drove home in shocked silence. It was when the explanatory literature arrived that the hopeless reality hit home, and Dot describes that day as the most frightening and hurtful day of her life.

Furthermore, Dot was advised to become sterilised, as it was believed then that subsequent children were bound to be CF sufferers and more seriously affected. We now know this is not the case, and genetic screening helps parents to make informed choices. It is difficult to imagine the feelings of utter devastation at this time. Dot was facing the eventual loss of her only child and the prospect of never becoming a mother. Her life plan was shattered.

Meanwhile the priority was making sure that Christine received the best available treatment. They lived with the uncertainty of the condition, swinging between hope and crisis, but determined that Christine would beat the system. A lot of research into CF was going on in the seventies and eighties, so that Christine became part of an educative process for the medical staff who cared for her. Although a lot more is now known about the illness, there is still no cure.

Dot feels that Christine dealt with her illness better than she did.

'She was great fun, strong, academically brilliant, a really steady girl who took everything in her stride. I would say to her, "I don't know how you are managing this", and she would say, "Well, this is happening to me, so you can't know as much as me about how I feel". You couldn't talk for her – she talked to the doctors for herself. They said she was a receptive and inquisitive patient, and she obviously built relationships with them. She told her consultant that she knew she was dying at least six months before she died. I was so impressed by the effect of her dying on other people, including the doctors and nurses. She amazed me that she behaved with such dignity.'

Christine was 13 when she died.

'It was a time of absolute devastation. Everything about our lives had been easy and happy – and then this was the first real challenge we had to face on our own and could not overcome. It was the end of the dream of having children and being a family. So what future did we have now? I had lost my identity. Although surrounded by family and friends, it felt like we were left with nothing.'

But Dot had been left with something very important, from Christine herself. When she had only hours to live, and both knew it, Dot asked Christine what she could do for her. Christine replied, 'Help other children and their parents'.

'It was like she was saying, don't just give up – do something to make things easier for other people. Living with a terminal illness took nothing away from her concern for others, and this was something I noticed in her which I didn't see in myself. She made me aware that other people were suffering too and she taught me to be more unselfish. This is one of the gifts she gave to me and why I'm so proud of her. So when she died, I needed to help others or I would be letting her down.'

The opportunity for helping others came with an approach from the medical staff who tried to keep Christine alive, but had begun to realise that their work with the parents was not finished when the child died. As Dot had asked Christine, so now the hospital asked Dot, 'What can we do for you?' She was able to say that she wanted the support that comes from being able to talk – to go over it all again with medical staff, and to share experiences with other bereaved parents. She was invited to join a new Bereavement Group at Alder Hey Hospital, whose efforts culminated in setting up the Alder Centre. She became a tireless fundraiser and developed the skills for supporting more recently bereaved parents.

> 'I couldn't take their pain away, but I understood their need to talk. Helping to give people a place to talk in and people to talk to became my therapy. And then there came the realisation that we needed to think bigger, to build the resources of the Centre, to have the help of professionals for those who needed more than just talking.'

Dot found herself in demand to speak at conferences, to raise awareness of the needs of bereaved families.

> 'I had to dig deep to find the resources to stand up in front of people and talk to them. That was really hard to start with, but friends encouraged me to believe I could do it. Suddenly I was the expert, because I had lost a child. I have gone out and done things I wouldn't do normally, because I knew how proud of me Christine would be if I stuck at it. Everything I have done for bereavement support has been in her name.'

Looking back, Dot never thought there could ever be any positive meaning coming from Christine's death. But that has changed.

> 'There's never a day goes by that I don't wake in the morning and think of her, but not always in a sad way now. She's my driving force, even 25 years down the line and even though my life has changed a lot. I have been very positive in accepting what I can do, and she gave me the strength to do these things. I also have the backing of good friends who still talk about her. There is nothing negative now. Christine's death was inevitable, and she was born to die at an early age. At times I can still slide back, on anniversaries for example, but now I can handle myself with more dignity and feel better

for it. I feel very honoured that Christine was in my life, and I came to that conclusion quite early on.'

DOREEN AND RICHARD

15 April 1989: the date of the football disaster at Hillsborough Stadium, Sheffield, when Liverpool were drawn against Nottingham Forest in the FA Cup semi-final. Ninety-six Liverpool fans were crushed to death as a result of police mismanagement of the crowd. Among the dead were Doreen's elder son Richard, aged 25, and his girlfriend Tracy. They were both studying and living together in Sheffield. Doreen's daughter Stephanie, at 18 her first time at an away match, survived. She had become separated from her brother and suffered the trauma of waiting at the side of the pitch, with other injured and disorientated fans, for Richard to find her.

Back in Liverpool, Doreen became aware of 'trouble' at the match from media coverage and then from a public phone call from a distressed Stephanie (no mobile phones then). Doreen and Leslie, her husband, travelled to Sheffield that evening, hoping and believing that Richard and Tracy would be among the injured in hospital. They were taken to the Boys' Club, which was being used as an emergency rest centre, where bewildered social workers and priests attempted to support anxious families. Doreen and Leslie were taken to the football ground to look at photographs of those who had died. After they found Richard and Tracy, two zipped body bags were brought to them for identification. Doreen wanted to touch Richard but was not allowed to. She was told, 'These bodies belong to the coroner now'.

After giving statements, which included answering questions about Richard's drinking habits and their own drinking habits, they were reunited with Stephanie and went with a priest to Richard and Tracy's flat before driving home. Two days later they returned to Sheffield, as Doreen was still desperate to touch and hold Richard's body. She was only permitted to see his body through glass. When eventually his body was brought back to Liverpool a week later for the funeral, it was too late for Doreen to touch him as she longed to do.

Doreen was left with a sense of outrage, for themselves, that they should have been treated with such little respect, and for Richard, that he was treated as a criminal or a hooligan. Early police statements clearly blamed the fans for the tragedy, saying that they had arrived for the match late and drunk and had forced open a gate. The truth, which later emerged, was that police had opened an exit gate to allow supporters to enter together, rather than singly through turnstiles. Although the central pens at the Leppings Lane entrance were already full, there was no police direction to the side pens where there was still room. As soon as the supporters entered the terraces they were swept off their feet and forced against steel barriers and the pitch-side fencing. Those at the front desperately appealed to security guards and police for help, but their shouting was misinterpreted as aggression and their calls were ignored until it was too late.

No wonder, then, that the grieving families felt betrayed by those who should have protected them. Those early police lies were compounded by scurrilous reports in *The Sun* newspaper that Liverpool fans had picked the pockets of the dead and urinated on their bodies. The hurt and anger felt by the families energised the formation of the Hillsborough Families' Support Group, who led calls for a public inquiry. The families are still outraged that, after Lord Justice Taylor's official inquiry clearly exposed the police cover-up, after a lengthy inquest, high court appeals and a judicial process of scrutiny, no-one has ever been found accountable.

Doreen, who was devastated by Richard's death, joined the Families' Support Group. The Group brought relief that she was not alone with her unanswered questions and anger. Doreen's involvement with the Group gave her the will to fight.

'At the time of Richard's death, all I could feel was utter devastation. I couldn't imagine my life without him, I didn't want my life without him. I had been an outgoing person, but now I became frightened of people, and even thought of taking my own life. I couldn't stop crying. But in time I just had to get up and live every day, I had to change my life, and try to find someone in myself I could live with. The old Doreen had gone and wasn't coming back, and I didn't like the person I had become. So I changed things. I started walking, I started writing poetry, I left my office job for a job working with the blind, and I got involved with the legal side of the Hillsborough Families' Support Group.

Richard had given me so much, and I wanted to give something back, something I could do for other people. I wanted to find a forum for saying how bereaved parents should and should not be treated. I was able to do that through my voluntary work, first for the Hillsborough Group and then for the Alder Centre.'

Doreen holds her memory of Richard with great pride. She describes him as physically attractive, with footballing 'thunder thighs'; as being passionately interested in the environment and geology; as a postgraduate student in chemistry with a bright research future; and as a generous and decent human being.

> 'I had him for 25 years and feel very positive about that. The memory of the joy he brought me runs alongside the pain of his not being here. I can still feel very vulnerable, and you scratch the surface and I'm back in touch with the distress. But I have learnt ways to protect myself, especially when talking to the media. I have now found a person inside myself that I can live with.
>
> The voluntary work I do to support other bereaved parents is a tribute to Richard. I can reassure them that while the pain does not go away, you can learn to live with it. Richard was my eldest, and he was my learning curve. There is nothing positive in his death, though there are positives which have come from his death.
>
> I have a good life now, and I adore my grandchildren. My grandson aged 13 recently told me, "My dad had a brother you know . . . and when my dad tells me more about him I will let you know."
>
> Richard is always on my mind, and forever in my heart. I believe I will see him again one day, and that's a great comfort.'

BARBARA AND DANIEL

Barbara's first child, Daniel, was born in 1992. Her instinct that there was 'something not right' was borne out when Daniel stopped breathing one day when he was six months old. After hospital tests he was diagnosed as a Fallot Baby with pulmonary stenosis, that is, he had a hole in his heart and narrowing of the arteries. Corrective surgery was planned for two years old, but at 12 months Daniel's condition deteriorated and the surgery was brought forward and took place when he was 14 months old. Barbara and her husband Wayne were told there was a 95% chance of survival, so they could be confident of success. However, Daniel came out of theatre in a very poorly condition, and died the following day, which was Mother's Day.

> 'I would say now I'm a very positive person, but at that time I sort of knew

he wouldn't make it. Preparing myself for the worst then turned into guilt, because I should have been more optimistic. The guilt was worse because, even though I was brought up a Roman Catholic, I had Daniel baptised by a friendly Church of England vicar – so I felt punished for not having him baptised as a Catholic.'

Barbara describes the disintegration of her identity in stark terms:

'One day I was Daniel's mum, and the next day I was worthless and redundant. I had totally lost my position, felt alienated from everyone, and didn't belong anywhere. Wayne had his job to go back to, and I resented that. I was very wrapped up in myself and felt no-one cared. Everything had lost its meaning and purpose. I didn't wash, I didn't change my clothes often enough, I didn't do any housework. I drove around without tax and insurance because I was so angry with everything and everyone.

The cemetery became my life. I used to spend up to eight hours a day in the cemetery in the days following the funeral, partly because I felt Daniel was there and I was with him, and partly because I was looking for other children's graves and wanted to meet other parents who had lost a child. After five days I did meet another bereaved mother. We clung together, and used to have "sit-ins" in the cemetery, because once I walked through those cemetery gates, I felt more balanced and okay. His death had consumed my life, just as his life had, so I had nothing else to focus on.'

James was born prematurely seven months after Daniel died. Barbara remembers little of his early years, and didn't allow herself to enjoy him until he was four or five years old. She still lives with the fear of losing James, and can never take him for granted. The positive which comes from that is the close and open relationship they now have.

Looking back, Barbara can actually feel grateful for the experience of being a bereaved parent.

'Now I am glad – and this sounds really awful – to have experienced what I have. Of course I'd rather have Daniel back, but I have a sense of becoming a totally different person than I would have been, having gone through those pain barriers. I have a far better tolerance and understanding, I know what is and isn't important, and I have a different way of seeing people. It has been important to do things in his memory to help others – especially when newly bereaved parents think they're going mad or want to kill themselves. Becoming a befriending volunteer at the Alder Centre and getting involved in the Centre's growth are really important to me. Wayne and I started by learning from other parents' experience, and now we can contribute to helping others. Also, in my work as a family court officer, I can feel empathy for parents who "lose" their children through custody arrangements.

Daniel may only have lived for 14 months, but he has lived within me for 18 years, and we both take him forward with us. We have continued to talk about him and his memory has never faded. It's just that his purpose has changed over the years. I believe he supports me, like a spiritual guide. When times are hard and I go down again, I feel him there saying, "Come on, you can do this".

Something that Barbara has been able to do has been in the face of an almost unbelievable twist of fate. In September 1999 Barbara and Wayne were informed that Daniel had been one of the children whose organs had been retained for research purposes without their knowledge at Alder Hey Hospital. First they were told that only his heart had been taken, then that all his organs had been retained, including his eyes. Then, having at last buried his organs in 2007, they were told a year later that a ghastly mistake had occurred. What they had buried included some of Daniel's organs together with some organs from another child.

'We felt hammered, constantly knocked back down, and I went into meltdown for a while. When we first heard about the organs, we were devastated, let down, angry and bitter. For a while we became obsessed with asking questions and trying to find answers, so that in the end we had to make a conscious decision to move away from that. Some of the parents affected formed a group, but we didn't join them because their attitudes were so negative and destructive. We fell back on the support of the friends we had made through the Alder Centre, and I had to ask myself, "How can I fight the hospital I am supporting?"

Then I was invited to join a Steering Group set up by the hospital to develop procedures for the disposal of unclaimed body parts. What gave me the strength to do this? I actually gained a sense of privilege from seeing those unclaimed organs, and thinking I could have a part in helping to oversee the respectful burials planned for them. It was like Daniel was saying, "There you go, you need to be a part of helping to sort this out".

The strength of my marriage has helped me throughout, and we have a real sense of partnership. Recently our 25th wedding anniversary provided the opportunity for celebrating that partnership with good friends who help us feel rich.'

JOHN AND JENNY

John describes his daughter Jenny as a very kind and caring girl who, as a teenager, was more interested in fundraising for the 'Give every child a chance' campaign than dressing up and going out. Jenny was seven years old when her parents divorced, but John continued to be actively involved in her care. He gave up his engineering work on offshore rigs for a job nearer to home so that he could be more available as a father. When Jenny became pregnant at 17 and the father of the baby disappeared off the scene, all the family pulled together to support her, and the plan was for John to buy a flat to share with Jenny and her baby. In the first weeks after Jonathon's birth, John took Jenny and the baby out with great pride. John was only 39 and remembers people assuming he was the baby's father rather than his grandfather.

Jenny was killed when Jonathon was only seven weeks old. She had been cycling to a friend's house when she was hit by a truck, and there was nothing on her person to enable the police to identify her. John had driven past the build-up of traffic at the accident scene unaware that Jenny was involved . . . but when he discovered that she had not arrived at her friend's house he phoned the police, to be told that a young woman answering her description had been taken to hospital. Jenny had suffered brain damage and was unconscious, and John recalls his surprise that there was not a mark on her.

John stayed at Jenny's bedside for five days until all hope was lost for her recovery and her life support was switched off.

What did Jenny's death mean to John?

'I just saw my future and Jenny's future and Jonathon's future with Jenny disappear into a kind of blackness. We had all these plans – Jenny was going to do hairdressing and beauty – she absolutely doted on Jonathon, and was going to be a fantastic mother. So it was an enormous loss. The future looked bleak. Trying to find words to express the pain of losing a child is so difficult.

I guess a big part came out in my behaviour at that time: I used to get very angry and when I played five-a-side football I used to pick on the biggest fellas and was frightened of no-one. I had a complete change of personality and had all these feelings coming up that I couldn't put words to. When these feelings sneaked up on me I thought, "My God, how do I respond to this?" It was a massive learning curve during the first few years after she died, having to adapt to new emotions and experiences.'

John can point to a couple of things that helped him to cope. First, there was his four-year-old son Marc from a relationship subsequent to his divorce, although this relationship too had broken down. John got his flat and had Marc to stay, and Marc insisted that John play football with him and helped him regain some motivation. Baby Jonathon also came to stay and the three of them would go out for the day.

'Just being with them helped me focus on what was important in my life now. The two fellas needed me to be functioning. They gave my life some meaning.'

Secondly, he joined a support group for bereaved parents at the Alder Centre, which John found extremely helpful. He remains passionate about the value of such groups, which he now helps to run himself.

There followed a time of transition that transformed John's life and culminated in John becoming a professionally qualified counsellor. Twelve months after joining the group he noticed changes in himself:

'I realised I was coping better and relating to people better. I didn't know what was happening, but something was.'

A couple of years later John volunteered for the Helpline at the Alder Centre, which left him eager to learn more about using his experience to support others. He went on to sign up for a certificate in counselling, all the while developing a new language for what he knew instinctively. Looking back, he understood his use of empathy when 'macho' men on the construction sites had talked to him about their problems. He wanted to devote himself to a new career, and dropped his engineering work to complete a counselling diploma and move on to a job at the Alder Centre as a counsellor and helping to train new volunteers.

'The counselling training made me see qualities in myself I didn't know were there. Jenny's death was the catalyst for that. Who knows whether I would have found my way to this new direction anyway, but she certainly speeded up the process. Now, at an age when I should be looking at retiring, I still want to learn more. I wonder if people look at me and think I might be answering a need in myself to be working as a counsellor to bereaved parents, but I don't think so. I can manage to keep my own grief separate, and I believe my resilience has strengthened over the years.'

Who or what has helped John to build that resilience? First and foremost, John recognises the importance of a good support network, which now includes his current partner and their young son Joe.

'I made sure that I spent time with people whom I cared about and who cared about me. I was very selective about what information I shared with other people when I was feeling vulnerable, until I felt stronger. In other words, I learned to look after myself. The worst thing that could ever happen has happened and I have survived. My priorities have changed as a result, which means I can invest in new relationships and family life.'

COLIN AND TIM

On Saturday, 20 March 1993, two bombs concealed in litterbins exploded in Bridge Street, Warrington. Two boys, Tim Parry, aged 12 and Johnathan Ball, aged 3, died as a result of the blasts. Fifty-six other people were injured. Tim, not usually an early riser, wanted to get into town to buy Everton goalkeeper shorts, having discovered a latent talent for keeping goal. Tim's parents, Colin and Wendy, have never been able to establish why Warrington was a target for this terrorist act. Warnings of attacks had been issued in Liverpool and Manchester but no warning had been issued for Warrington.

Colin had kept a daybook for each of his three children, recording key events in their lives from their birth, so his recollection of Tim's brief life is vivid.

'I am not going to sanctify my son. Tim had his own charm; he was a very social animal, more so than his older brother and his younger sister. Tim was the joker in the pack; he was very good at bringing people together and he was never, ever, in the house; he was always out. On the downside, his humour could be extremely rude, as you can imagine with boys at that age, and he could wind his older brother up something rotten, so Dominic would clobber him and I would have to separate them. Tim's character? On one level, gregarious, humorous, good fun, but he could be an antagonistic little sod who would drive his brother mad . . . two characters in one. Yet anything he could get involved in, he would; any sport he could partake in, he would. An ordinary boy.'

Colin has often pondered the statistical likelihood of Tim being caught up in the bombing and coming to terms with its impact on him and the family. Only recently has he found out the full nature of the effect of the blast on Tim's body.

'It was an unbelievable shock . . . an unbelievable time; not just that he had lost his life, but the manner in which he had lost his life. It was not until about a year-and-a-half ago that we got a copy of the coroner's report. I sat down and started reading and had to stop . . . it was ripping me inside. The injuries he sustained were horrifying . . . we knew that he had been seriously injured as the whole of his head was bandaged, all the damage being to his face and head . . . that's where the shrapnel had hit him. From the neck down, there were only minor injuries. Knowing the nature of his death and the brutality of it was frankly impossible to comprehend. Why Warrington? Why that day? Why that place? Why that bin? Why was Tim standing here and not there . . . a foot either way . . .? It was impossible to understand. Unless you have lost a child, it is hard to explain.'

Colin and Wendy had to face the decision to switch the life support machine off after five days. They both had very different ways of handling that. Some insensitivity on outlining the process by the neurosurgeon meant that Colin alone held Tim's hand when he died. Gordon Wilson, whose daughter Marie had been killed in the Remembrance Day Bombing in Enniskillen, visited the family on the day of Johnathan Ball's funeral. He offered Colin and Wendy some advice on dealing with their grief.

'Be forgiving of each other when you grieve, because you will grieve at different times, in different ways. You mustn't sit in judgement on each other, and don't be hard on each other.'

Colin says that he did not think that was ever going to happen; but Gordon was proved right.

> 'There were days when I was not on full form, when I thought that she was not hurting as much as me, she is getting over this too well. Wendy is much more internal than me. I express my views more openly . . .'

Colin feels that time has made him less vulnerable. Key dates such as Tim's birthday, Christmas and the anniversary of the bombing have their effect. He says that he rarely feels raw. People contacted him following other atrocities, for example 9/11 and 7/7, and asked him if it took him back. Very few things take him back but occasionally a piece of music does. He did, for a time, have many photographs of Tim, enlarged and framed, all over the house. Wendy was never a great fan of that, so when they moved homes they were moved to his study. Colin also had audio tapes made of Tim's voice, which he would play in the car.

Tim's death has had a long and lasting impact and effect on the wider family. Colin had wanted his children to experience university life; neither of his surviving children did. Dominic has taken some time to settle, via a variety of jobs, to a current career as a skilled tradesman, and Abbi, who became very quiet, took another route with her life. Both now have children of their own, and having grandchildren around feels good for Colin and Wendy.

What is Tim's legacy? Colin would agree that his life was very different pre March 1993. He described it as exceedingly ordinary and 'bog standard'. He worked in Human Resources in Kirkby and spent much of his time in negotiation and collective bargaining with trades unions. He would say that he was never short of an opinion, no shrinking violet, and maybe that attitude and skill set served him well for the situation after Tim's death.

> 'I was not ever going to lie down and try to be rational and reasonable. I couldn't accept that he had been killed, and then just get on with my life. That was not an option. I would have gone slowly insane. I now had a campaign to be involved in and that was the difference between sanity and insanity. Fortunately, Wendy, who is not like me, has always supported me. That was important, because if she had said "No, I am not doing any of this", then I think we may have fallen apart.'

This determination not to allow Tim to fade into a recollection resulted in the founding of a charity to promote peace. Colin and Wendy began the charity in 1995 and started with the modest activity of connecting peace groups in Warrington, Ireland and Northern Ireland. Through a youth worker, they organised a youth exchange programme. Through various visits to Ireland, they met a number of peace organisations on both sides of the border and developed warm friendships. The results of the various exchanges were so impressive and rewarding that they both wanted to do more of it.

Colin gave up his job in 1998, became self-employed, thus giving him more time to try to build what had been a tiny charity, run from what had been Tim's bedroom, into something more ambitious. The political climate was also changing at that time and, in Mo Mowlem (at that time the Secretary of State for Northern Ireland), Colin and Wendy found someone who was very receptive to being involved. Mo, by knocking on the right doors and speaking to the right people, helped them raise the funds to create a Peace Centre in Warrington. Through a combination of factors, the initial modest plans grew into the impressive Peace Centre in Warrington. Over £3 million was raised, and now the Peace Centre runs many activities, projects and programmes with the theme of building harmonious communities. The Centre carries the names of both Tim and Johnathan Ball.

(*See* the Tim Parry/Johnathan Ball Foundation for Peace www.foundation 4peace.org for further information.)

Postscript:
The IRA announced that from midnight on 31 August 1994 it would cease its campaign of terror.

> 'So, from the first minute of 1 September 1994, the day Tim would have been 14, the violence that took his life and vitality from us would be over. This was a poignant vindication that Tim did not die in vain. Six weeks later, on 13 October, the Loyalist paramilitaries declared their own ceasefire: the day after Dominic's 16th and Abbi's 13th birthdays. So again, it seemed that Tim was laying his own hand on events.'

DAVE AND CAROL AND A

Over the 15 years since Dave and Carol were approved as foster carers, they have cared for 96 children – some for a day, some for years – three of whom had life-limiting conditions and died while in their care.

They started while both were still in work, Dave full-time as a factory worker and Carol part-time as a carer in adult services. They talk about 'stumbling into' fostering, though they had talked about fostering 'one day' when their children, then 11 and eight, were older. In the event, when a social worker spotted Carol's ability for settling a fractious baby whose mother was in respite care, she told Carol: 'You really should foster – you're a natural – phone this number'. Carol did phone the fostering service and a 'Skills to Foster' course was due to start that same evening. It was as if it was meant to be.

They involved their children from the beginning and took them to every meeting as part of their preparation, and the children were 'totally on board with it'.

Dave and Carol were unsure what they could offer, but they had no hesitation in taking on disabled children. How did they develop this confidence to accept disability? Both came from big families and lost a parent at an early age, and point to these experiences as giving them a natural empathy with disadvantaged children. They also felt fortunate to have two healthy children themselves and their lifestyle was totally child-orientated. Dave speaks for both of them when he says:

> 'We have never looked at the child's disability, and always treated the child as a child. Different children have different disabilities and some of these can't be seen. A lot of people don't understand if they can't see a wheelchair.'

'A' was the first disabled child to stay with them permanently and he died after eleven-and-a-half years in their care. Meningitis as a baby had left him with profound disabilities. At first they had him for respite care at weekends, but had him full-time when his birth family could no longer care for him and the social worker could not find a suitable placement. On hearing this news and without thinking about it, Carol's response was, 'For goodness sake, build us an extension and we'll have him!'

This commitment confirmed Dave's decision to take early redundancy from his work to become A's principal carer, which turned out to be a 24-hour job. At every hospital appointment, the consultant was amazed to see A, as he wasn't expected to live beyond a year. In fact he lived until he was fourteen-and-a-half.

Dave and Carol talk about A with huge affection and respect. Carol describes A as 'one of the most charming young men you could ever wish to meet'. They recall his achievements with pride and humour.

> 'Other people would see these as very small improvements, but to us they were massive. Through a lot of encouragement he did eventually manage to grab a cup – though he couldn't always find his mouth!'

They were both tuned in to the sounds he made and he could communicate his feelings quite well without speech. Dave and Carol worked closely with the school he attended, which was very supportive. They chuckle about the day when A won an award for being the 'cheeriest child in the school'.

> 'He was just yelling for England and we just sat there in total awe of him. He knew everyone was making a fuss of him because he'd done something nice.'

How did they cope with knowing A would die? Carol explained:

> 'It was always there in the background, but we concentrated on having fun with him day by day. When he did die, it still took us both by surprise, because of how quickly he deteriorated. He had developed a chest infection, no different from previous occasions, but this time the antibiotics didn't work. We phoned his mother from the hospital and she came straight away. We had a wonderful relationship with her, and she always said that A had two mums and two dads . . . and she visited most weekends. When A died a few hours after his hospital admission, it was the most awful experience. Dave was at home going frantic but couldn't come because of looking after another child we had at the time. A's death was devastating for both of us, because whatever happened he always bounced back . . .'

As the main carer, Dave was the one who went to the hospital to dress him.

Dave and Carol had expected the Chinese birth family to want a traditional Chinese Buddhist funeral, but his birth mother insisted that he was to have the funeral that Dave and Carol wanted for him. They met together to arrange the funeral, and Buddhist officiants came to the funeral parlour to perform their traditional rites before the Christian service and cremation.

Everyone was invited to come to the funeral in brightly coloured clothes as a reflection of his life.

What did his death mean to Dave and Carol? Dave says:

'I can't put it into words how hard it was to lose him. I couldn't help thinking, did we do anything wrong, did we act quickly enough?'

Carol describes it as leaving a 'massive hole'.

'We felt empty . . . we went from doing everything for him to doing nothing . . . we were wandering round the house, and we were wondering whether we could do this again . . .

I might have been A's foster carer. But I couldn't have loved him any more if I had given birth to him. With A we willingly crossed the line from foster carers to foster parents. His birth parents gave us permission to be his parents too, so there was no fostering barrier there.

But in general we know we are foster carers, and obviously the birth parents have to be accommodated before us, and we have to take a step back. We knowingly do this, to care for a child with a life-limiting condition, whereas the birth parents don't have a choice.'

So had this experience of losing A made them more vulnerable or more resilient? Carol's response:

'At first we said, we can't do this again – but we did, and we got through it.

After we lost A, he never let us give up on anyone. Later, a consultant for a life-limited child we were caring for warned us that we would get nothing from looking after this child. I thought, that's not for you to say.

I think he could only see the disability and the limitations, and couldn't see past that – but it's not only about what they can do physically, it's what you get back emotionally.'

Dave's response:

'He taught us such a lot . . . he was that loving and that giving he just beamed . . . And I believe that A did everything he wanted to do and got fulfilment from everything he did.

He taught us that, as long as you look for another route, anything is possible. We both believe that everybody deserves a chance, no matter what colour, nature, culture . . . At the end of the day these children were put on this earth for a reason, and they should be given every chance to develop their potential.'

So what enables Dave and Carol to care for children with such extreme disabilities? Carol and Dave are used to finishing each others' sentences, and both readily acknowledge that their relationship is key, that after 30 years they are still best friends and they work well as partners. They are both comfortable with tears and with each other's emotions. Whatever the challenge, Carol says:

'As long as I can acknowledge I am struggling, then I know I can get through it. I have never lost passion for what we do'.

And Dave has the last word:

'Looking back I wouldn't do anything different. I never regretted finishing work, where I was just a number. Now I know I have made a difference.'

ANNE AND OSCAR

Oscar was born in August 2001 with an unusual congenital malformation: a dark brown birthmark covering his buttocks, thighs and part of his back, which was a huge shock to his parents, Anne and Martin. At first the main concern was one of aesthetics, since they were told there was only a 1% chance that this could become cancerous. However, seven months later a biopsy confirmed the development of a melanoma, and at a year old, Oscar had surgery followed by chemotherapy to deal with a lump in his groin. Six months later another lump in his other groin led to further surgery, and by December the disease had progressed to the point that the hospital doctors told Anne and Martin that nothing more could be done for Oscar. They brought him home, where he died two weeks before Christmas, aged two years and four months.

Right up to those last two weeks Oscar had remained a vibrant and happy child, who constantly challenged the medical norms for recovery. Anne describes him as having a strong, engaging personality.

'He was just such a bright little boy. I remember when he was born he looked all-knowing, and I know it sounds daft, but I had this feeling right from the start that he knew what was going on, but he was going to do his own thing anyway!

He was walking at nine months, and you could have a good conversation with him by the time he was two years old. I know every parent thinks their child is bright, but he really was, and others saw it too.

He was a joy, an absolute joy. He was such good company, and entertaining. When he walked into a room full of people, he worked the room, interacting with everyone in turn. He loved people and seemed interested in everything. He was emotionally intelligent too, and would pick up on others' feelings. Once when we were on the hospital ward, being given some bad news by the consultant, he looked up and said to us, "I love you so much", as if he knew we were hurting.'

Anne has no doubt that Oscar lived his life to the full, and that the quality of his life cannot be measured by how long he lived.

'I have this sense that although his life was short, it was still his whole life, and he lived every minute as "pure Oscar". I get some comfort from that, knowing that he never learned to modify his behaviour to please others.'

So what did his death mean to Anne?

'Everything. I felt like my whole life had come to a standstill. He was the focus of my life, so his death left a huge, huge hole. I was still his mother, but I no longer had the role of his mother. Initially the physical loss was just too much, and I couldn't deal with it. It took three to four years before the reality sunk in and I could talk about Oscar without getting overwhelmed.

But at the same time I never felt that he had left me. I very soon started writing to Oscar in my journal, telling him about my day and how much I missed him. In a sense I could still hear him and we were still having a relationship. I don't write so much now, but I still talk to him in my head and include him in my life.

Whenever I felt desperate in those early days I was reassured by remembering him singing the words to "Going on a Bear Hunt": "You can't get over it, you can't go under it, you can't go round it – you just have to go through it".'

At first Anne oscillated between being vulnerable to those desperate feelings and drawing on her inner resources to keep going. Looking back she can see an overall progression towards becoming more resilient, though she can still go backwards.

> 'I will always get upset thinking about Oscar's death, but then I remember that he is still with me – not physically, but he is in my heart and forever part of me. The essence of him is not a physical thing, and his energy lives on. It's like the first law of thermodynamics: "Energy cannot be created or destroyed – it just changes from one form to another".'

Clearly Anne has no problem in seeing meaning in Oscar's life, but what about meaning and purpose in her own life since he died?

> 'There has to be some degree of hope in order to carry on. Although I often lost sight of that hope in the early days, I always had the hope – tested hugely as time went on – that I would become a mother again one day. And I always believed that Oscar was something quite special, so that even if I didn't become a mother again, even if that's all I ever do, and the rest of my life is uneventful, then that was enough . . .'

Happily, on the last day of 2008, after five years of trying for another baby, Oscar's twin brothers Felix and Jasper were born. It helped Anne to know she was having twins, as she knew that neither could be a replacement for Oscar. Anne's hope and resilience have won through.

> 'I am only here today because of everything that's happened and everyone I have met. In terms of resilience, I don't like phrases such as "come to terms with" and "moving on". Basically life goes on. When you lose a child it shakes you to the core and everything falls apart. You have to rebuild yourself, but with the new reality that your child has died. You have to accept that's happened and incorporate it into your new life and it becomes part of you. You don't move on and leave things behind, because you take them with you. Oscar is still part of my life.'

COMMENT

The observations that follow come from Gail Ashton, a colleague in the counselling world, who can comment both from personal experience and from her research findings involving other bereaved mothers. From this research she wrote an article, 'Pebble on My Wing', published in *Therapy Today*, reflecting on the potential for 'growth from adversity'. Her comments bring together the personal and professional, combine theory with experience, and reflect key concepts in the development of our understanding of what it means to lose a child.

'My story, which led eventually to the research for my MA dissertation, began 15 years ago when my youngest son Sam died suddenly and traumatically, at the age of five, whilst we were on holiday in France. Our son Tom (then aged seven) also witnessed his little brother's death. I was at that time an art teacher, and three years later decided to change direction and train as a counsellor/psychotherapist. I worked in primary care for two years and then decided to integrate my clinical experience and educational experience and began working in higher education as a counsellor.

For my Masters research dissertation I explored the experiences of other bereaved mothers. Whilst I would have wanted to explore fathers' and siblings' grief too, it was a small-scale study and needed to be limited and focused. The research study explored the grief experience of bereaved mothers after the death of their child and considered how or whether their world view was changed, how they rebuilt "self" while adapting to a new and changed life, and explored the importance of the value of remaining connected to and continuing the bond with their child. As a bereaved mother I remained visible within the research, integrating my own personal and professional experience alongside the stories of the research participants.

For many bereaved parents their view of the world and assumptions about safety, security, predictability, and trust are understandably challenged and changed. The death of a child contradicts the perceived natural order of life, violating and shattering the parents' assumptive world. We do not expect our children to die before their parents and grandparents. Bereaved parents and siblings experience a sense of unjustness and unfairness, which can challenge the basis of all previously held beliefs and assumptions about self, life and the world. Many bereaved parents describe how the death of their child opens up the possible vulnerability and fragility of others whom they love, becoming fearful for other family members and feeling vulnerable and sensitive to the possibility of further life tragedies. However, such a challenge can also create an existential crisis, a search for the meaning of what it is to be human and a search to make sense of the death of their child and to find some important existential benefit or life lesson.

I had experienced such a change of my life view some years after the death of Sam. I had begun to experience a determination, eagerness and passion to enjoy life and those relationships in my life which I valued. Reordering my priorities and even changing my profession was part of that shift. I noticed that where once I would hesitate to do things, I began to be more spontaneous and sometimes adventurous. Things which were once very important to me, such as routines and self-expectations, became less important to me and instead, valuing, cherishing, and enjoying life in the moment became more of a focus.

I became aware that partly I wanted to live my life in memory of and for Sam, and partly I wanted to live it for me too. Not only had I "lost" my son, but I had also lost a part of myself when he died, and as the years passed I began to experience a sadness that Sam could not live his life further, and also a compassion for myself as a bereaved mother, and I felt determined and excited about the prospect of living for both of us. I also realised how, at any moment, any one of us can die. It is the one certainty from the day we are born, and somehow knowing the fact of death experientially and **viscerally**, and therefore more sharply after the death of a child, can spur one to live life in a more urgent and vivid way.

My research found that the bereaved mothers I interviewed had also experienced significant changes in self and attitudes such as a new enthusiasm for living, pride in self, contentment, strength, confidence, and a new sense of enrichment, joy, and pleasure alongside the continuing pain of loss and an ongoing relationship with the child. The notion of the benefits for the bereaved of continuing their relationship with the person who has died is relatively new, and emerged strongly within this research as vital to healthy grieving for all.

When I interviewed the bereaved mothers for my research dissertation, I felt moved and inspired by their lives, and how they had negotiated what is the bleakest of landscapes. It is a very lonely place in the context of the 21st century to be a bereaved parent or sibling. In the not too distant past, mortality in children and adults was higher, and there would have been a natural understanding of grief and particularly child death borne out of familiarity. Thankfully today, it is less common. However, it can now mean that bereaved families feel more isolated and they do not have the support mechanisms which come from an experience being commonplace and familiar. Bereaved parents in the 21st century can therefore feel very isolated, alone, and separate from others and society and many will find solace with other bereaved parents through bereaved parent groups or support organisations.

What was incredibly moving, inspiring, and uplifting about the findings of this research was the way the bereaved mothers articulated their love for their children, their ongoing grief, their continuing relationship with their child, and also the hopeful changes in their lives since the trauma of their losses.

I believe both personally and professionally that one of the reasons why the bereaved mothers I interviewed had been able to move forward in a hopeful way was because they allowed themselves to remain connected to their children and continue the bond with them.

The assumption that trauma always results in disorder should not be replaced with expectations that growth is inevitable either, and equally the unhelpful and rather hopeful idea that "good comes out of bad" or that "every cloud has a silver lining". It is a fact that life does carry on, as certainly as one day follows the next, even though for many bereaved parents they might wish it could just stop. However it is necessary for life to continue and for parents to find a way of doing that, which still holds the pain of loss of the child and the knowledge that they lived and died alongside a realisation that life is short, precious, and to be lived.'

Realising that 'life is short, precious, and to be lived' is something that comes to most of us late in life, when faced by our own mortality. Perhaps the child who dies leaves the gift of teaching us how to live our lives to the full.

The parents who have contributed to this chapter have left a message more powerful than anything I could write. Their contributions have touched me deeply and made me realise that we must all live our lives as best we can in the full knowledge that we too will die.

References

Ashton G. Pebble on my wing. *Therapy Today*. Lutterworth: BACP; June 2007.

Cyrulnik B. *Resilience: how your inner strength can set you free from the past*. London: Penguin; 2009.

Joseph S, Linley PA. *Positive Therapy. A meta-theory for positive psychological practice*. London: Routledge; 2006.

Machin L. Resilience in bereavement: Part 1. In: Monroe B, Oliviere D, editors. *Resilience in Palliative Care.* Oxford: Oxford University Press; 2007. pp. 157–165.

Yalom I. *Staring at the Sun: overcoming the dread of death.* London: Piatkus; 2008.

Further reading

Machin L. *Working with Loss and Grief.* Thousand Oaks, CA: Sage Publications; 2009.

Parry C, Parry W. *Tim: An Ordinary Boy.* London: Coronet Books; 1994.

Useful contacts for support organisations

The organisations listed below are either mentioned in the text or have a concern to support bereaved families and/or professionals.

Acorns Children's Hospice Trust

As well as providing home support, respite and terminal care, Acorns offers long-term bereavement support for families and a comprehensive training programme.

Acorns Children's Hospice Trust
Drakes Court
Alcester Road
Wythall
Birmingham B47 6JR

Tel: 0121 248 4850
www.acorns.org.uk

ACT (Association for Children with life-threatening or Terminal conditions and their families)

Umbrella organisation providing information about available services.

Brunswick Court
Brunswick Square
Bristol BS2 8PE

Tel: 0117 916 6422   Helpline: 0845 108 2201
www.act.org.uk   Email: info@act.org.uk

Alder Centre

For *all* those affected by the death of a child, providing support and counselling for families, and information and training for professionals.

Royal Liverpool Children's NHS Trust
Alder Hey
Eaton Road
Liverpool L12 2AP

Tel: 0151 252 5391   Helpline: 0800 282986
www.alderhey.com   Email: aldercentre@yahoo.co.uk

ARC (Ante-natal Results and Choices)

Information to parents and professionals and national helpline and befriending service.

73 Charlotte Street
London W1T 4PN

Tel: 020 7631 0285 (Helpline); 020 7631 0280 (Administration)
Email: info@arc-uk.org

Association for Children with Heart Disorders

Support for families with children suffering from heart disorders.

26 Elizabeth Drive
Helmshaw
Rossendale
Lancashire BB4 4JB

Tel: 01706 221988
Email: information@heartchild.info

Bliss

Support for families and carers of babies born prematurely or sick.

9 Holyrood Street
London SE1 2EL

Tel: 020 7378 1122
Helpline: 0500 618140
www.bliss.org.uk

British Association for Counselling and Psychotherapy (BACP)

Will help potential clients to find a suitable counsellor in their area.

BACP House
15 St John's Business Park
Lutterworth LE17 4HB

Tel: 01455 883300
www.bacp.co.uk   Email: bacp@bacp.co.uk

Childhood Bereavement Network (a National Children's Bureau charity)

National, multi-professional federation of organisations and individuals working with bereaved children and young people, providing an online directory, training and educational materials.

8 Wakley Street
London EC1 V 7QE

Tel: 020 7843 6309
www.childhoodbereavementnetwork.org.uk   Email: cbn@ncb.org.uk

Child Death Helpline

For all those affected by the death of a child, staffed by bereaved parents.
Every evening 7pm to 10pm, Monday to Friday 10am to 1pm
Tuesday and Wednesday 1pm to 4pm

Freephone: 0800 282986

CLIC Sargent

Caring for children with cancer.

Griffin House
161 Hammersmith Road
London W6 8SG

Offices also in Bristol, Belfast and Glasgow.

Tel: 020 8752 2800   Helpline: 0800 197 0068
www.clicsargent.org.uk   Email: helpline@clicsargent.org.uk

Compassionate Friends

Nationwide self-help organisation for bereaved parents and their families; resource library; advice leaflets; group and telephone support.

53 North Street
Bristol BS3 1EN

Tel: 0845 120 3785
Helpline: open every day 10am to 4pm, 6.30pm to 10.30pm,
  0845 123 2304
www.tcf.org.uk   Email: info@tcf.org.uk

Cruse Bereavement Care

Bereavement care provided by trained counsellors, plus advice and information on practical problems and befriending.

PO Box 800, Richmond
Surrey TW9 1RG

Tel: 020 8939 9530   Helpline: 0844 477 9400
www.crusebereavementcare.org.uk   Email: info@cruse.org.uk

Cystic Fibrosis Trust Research, support and education.

11 London Road
Bromley
Kent BR1 1BY

Tel: 020 8464 7211
www.cftrust.org.uk

Edward's Trust

Caring for families and children during child illness and bereavement.

43a Calthorpe Road
Edgbaston
Birmingham B15 1TS

Tel: 0121 456 4838
www.edwardstrust.org.uk   Email: admin@edwardstrust.org.uk

Foundation for the Study of Infant Deaths

Research, support, information and good practice guidelines.

11 Belgrave Road
London SW1V 1RB

Tel: 020 7802 3200; Helpline: Every day 6pm to 11pm
Monday to Friday 9am to 6pm, 020 7233 2090

www.fsid.org.uk   Email: office@fsid.org.uk

Hawthorn House: Yorkhill Family Bereavement Service

Providing a support and counselling service to anyone affected by the death
of a child, including support to children who have been bereaved.

Family Bereavement Service
Yorkhill NHS Trust
Glasgow G3 8SJ

Tel: 0141 201 9257
www.nhsggc.org.uk

ISIDA (Irish Sudden Infant Death Association)

Carmichael House
4 North Brunswick Street
Dublin 7

Tel: (outside Ireland) (00) 3531 873 2711
National Lo-call Helpline: 1850 391 391
Email: isida@eircom.net

Laura Centre

For *anyone* affected by the death of a child, providing professional counselling support and supervision.

4–6 Tower Street
Leicester LE1 6WS

Tel: 0116 254 4341
www.thelauracentre.org.uk   Email: info@thelauracentre.org.uk

Macmillan Cancer Support

Funds Macmillan nurses to give advice and support for cancer patients and their families.

89 Albert Embankment
London SE1 7UQ

Tel: 020 7840 7840   Helpline: 0808 800 1234
www.macmillan.org

Miscarriage Association

Provides support and information on pregnancy loss.

c/o Clayton Hospital
Northgate
Wakefield
West Yorkshire WF1 3JS

Tel: 01924 200795   Helpline: 01924 200795
www.miscarriageassociation.org.uk

National Association of Bereavement Services

Referral agency, information about services and training.

2nd floor
4 Pinchin Street
London E1 6DB

Tel: 020 7709 0505   Helpline: 020 7709 9090
www.stjohnshospice.org

PAPYRUS

National UK charity for the prevention of young suicide, providing resources and support for those affected.

HOPELineUK 08000 68 41 41
www.papyrus-uk.org

Sands (Stillbirth and Neonatal Death Society)

Supporting anyone affected by the death of a baby and promoting research to reduce the loss of babies' lives.

28 Portland Place
London W18 1LY

Tel: 020 7436 7940
www.uk-sands.org

Helpline Tel: 020 7436 5881
Email: support@uk-snads.org

Scottish Cot Death Trust

Research, support, information and good practice guidelines.

Royal Hospital for Sick Children
Yorkhill
Glasgow G3 8SJ

Tel: 0141 357 3946
www.sidscotland.org.uk

TAMBA (Twins And Multiple Births Association)

Provides information and mutual support networks for families of twins, triplets and more.

2 The Willows
Gardner Road
Guildford
Surrey GU1 4PG

Tel: 01483 304442
www.tamba.org.uk

TAMBA Twinline: 0800 138 0509
Email: Enquiries@tamba.org.uk

Winston's Wish

Charity for bereaved children and largest provider of services to bereaved families in the UK. Offers practical support and guidance to families, professionals, and anyone concerned about a grieving child.

Westmoreland House
80–6 Bath Road
Cheltenham
Glos GL53 7JT

Tel: 01242 515157
www.winstonswish.org.uk

Helpline: 08452 03 04 05
Email: info@winstonswish.org.uk

Children's hospices

Acorns for the Three Counties
350 Bath Road
Worcester WR5 3EZ
01905 767676   www.acorns.org.uk

Acorns in Birmingham
103 Oak Tree Lane
Selly Oak
Birmingham B29 6 Hz
0121 248 4850   www.acorns.org.uk

Acorns in the Black Country
Walstead Road
Walsall WS5 4LZ
01922 422500   www.acorns.org.uk

Bluebell Wood (The Richard Foundation)
Cramfit Road
North Anston
Sheffield S25 4AJ
0845 108 1579   www.bluebellwood.org

Brian House
Low Moor Road
Bispham
Blackpool FY2 0BG
01253 358881   www.brianhouse.inthefylde.org.uk

CHASE Hospice Care for Children
Loseley Park
Guildford
Surrey GU3 1HS
01483 454213   www.chasecare.org.uk

Chestnut Tree House
Dover Lane Poling
Arundel
West Sussex BN18 9PX
0845 450 5820   www.chestnut-tree-house.org.uk

Children's Hospice Association Scotland (Rachel House)
Avenue Road
Kinross KY13 8FX
01577 865777   www.chas.org.uk

Children's Hospice Association Scotland (Robin House)
2 Boturich Road
Balloch
Alexandria G83 8LX
01389 722055   www.chas.org.uk

Children's Hospice South West
Little Bridge House
Redlands Road
Fremington
North Devon EX31 2PZ
01271 325270   www.chsw.org.uk

Children's Hospice South West
Charlton Farm
Charlton Drive
Wraxall
North Somerset BS48 1PE
01275 866600   www.chsw.org.uk

Claire House
Clatterbridge Road
Bebington
Wirral CH63 4JD
0151 3430883   www.claire-house.org.uk

Demelza Hospice Care for Children
Rook Lane
Bobbing
Sittingbourne
Kent ME9 8DZ
01795 845200   www.demelzahouse.org.uk

Demelza Hospice Care for Children (Demelza James)
Red Lion House
Magham Down
Hailsham
East Sussex BN27 1PN
01323 446461   www.demelzahouse.org.uk

Demelza Hospice Care for Children (South London)
Wensley Close
Eltham
London SE9 5AB
020 8859 7766   www.demelzahouse.org.uk

Derian House
Chancery Road
Astley Village
Chorley
Lancashire PR7 1DH
01257 271271   www.derianhouse.org.uk

Donna Louise Children's Hospice
Treetops
1 Grace Road
Trentham
Stoke-on-Trent ST4 8TN
01782 654440   www.donnalouisetrust.org

East Anglia's Children's Hospices – Cambridge
Church Lane
Milton
Cambridge CB24 6AB
01223 205180   www.each.org.uk

East Anglia's Children's Hospices – Norfolk
Quidenhan
Norwich
Norfolk NR16 2PH
01953 715559   www.each.org.uk

East Anglia's Children's Hospices – Suffolk
6 Walker Close
Ipswich
Suffolk IP3 8LY
01473 714194   www.each.org.uk

Eden House
Durdar Road
Carlisle CA2 4SD
01228 817630   www.edenhouse.org.uk

Ellenor Shining lights
The Ellenor Centre
East Hill
Dartford
Kent DA1 1SA
01322 221315   www.lionshospice.co.uk

Francis House
390 Parrswood Road
East Didsbury
Manchester M9 8PB
0161 448 0255   www.francishouse.org.uk

Haven House Foundation
The White House
Mallinson Park
Woodford Green
Essex IG8 9lb
020 8505 9944   www.havenhouse.org.uk

Helen & Douglas House
14a Magdalen Road
Oxford
Oxon OX4 1RW
01865 794749   www.helenanddouglas.org.uk

Hope House
Nant Lane
Morda
Nr Oswestry
Shropshire SY10 9BX
01691 671671   www.hopehouse.org.uk

Horizon House
18 O'Neill Road
Newtownabbey
Belfast BT36 6WB
028 9077 7635   www.nihospice.org

Iain Rennie Hospice At Home
52a Western Road
Tring
Herts HP23 4BB
01442 890444   www.irhh.org

Julia's House Children's Hospice Service
Unit F1
Arena Business Centre
Holyrood Close
Poole
Dorset BH17 7FP
01202 607400   www.juliashouse.org

Keech Cottage
Great Bramingham Lane
Streatly
Luton
Bedfordshire LU3 3NT
01582 492339   www.pasque.org

Little Havens
Daws Heath Road
Thundersley
Benfleet
Essex SS7 2LH
01702 552200   www.littlehavens.org.uk

Martin House
Grove Road
Clifford
Wetherby LS23 6TX
01937 845045   www.martinhouse.org.uk

Naomi House
Stockbridge Road
Sutton Scotney
Winchester
Hants SO21 3JE
01962 760060   www.naomihouse.org.uk

Noah's Ark

Ganwick House
Wagon Road
Barnet
Herts EN4 0PH
0208 449 8877   www.noahsarkhospice.org.uk

Rainbows Children's Hospice

Lark Rise
off Hazel Road
Loughborough Leics LE11 2HS
01509 638000   www.rainbows.co.uk

Richard House Trust

Richard House Drive
London E16 3RG
020 7511 0222   www.richardhouse.org.uk

Shooting Star House

The Avenue, Hampton
Middlesex TW12 3RA
020 8783 2004   www.shootingstar.org.uk www.shooingstar.org.uk

St Andrew's Children's Hospice

Peaks Lane
Grimsby
North East Lincolnshire DN32 9RP
01472 350908   www.standrewshospice.com

St Oswald's Hospice

Regent Avenue
Gosforth
Newcastle-upon-Tyne NE3 1EE
0191 2850063   www.stoswalds.org.uk

The Butterwick Children's Hospice

Middlefield Road
Stockton-on-Tees TS19 8XN
01642 607748   www.butterwick.org.uk

The Jessie May Trust

35 Old School House
Kingswood Foundation Estate
Britannia Road
Kingswood
Bristol BS15 8DB
0117 958 2172   www.jessiemaytrust.org.uk

The West Yorkshire Forget Me Not Trust

Wellington Mills
Plover Road
Lindley
Huddersfield HD3 3h
01484 489789   www.forgetmenottrust.co.uk

Ty Gobaith

Tremorfa Lane
Groesnydd
Conwy LL32 8SS
01492 651900   www.tygobaith.org.uk

Ty Hafan

Hayes Road
Sully
Vale of Glamorgan CF64 5XX
02920 532200   www.tyhafan.org

Useful resources for working with children and families

Resource manuals and packs

Bayliss J. *Understanding Loss and Grief*. Cambridge: National Extension College; 1996.
Training pack for helping and caring professions.
Includes exercises correlated with NVQ tasks. Photocopiable.

Childhood Bereavement Network
Has produced a range of resources useful to schools and other organisations for young people, including a set of postcards *I can . . . You can . . .* to remind bereaved children and their carers of coping strategies. www.childhoodbereavementnetwork.org.uk

CRUSE. *Supporting Bereaved Children and Families*. London: Cruse-Bereavement Care; 1993.
A training manual.

Fabry L. *Death and Bereavement*. Milton Keynes: The Chalkface Project; 1995.
Photocopiable resource pack aimed at PSE or Religious Studies teachers.
Written by Fabry in consultation with Margaret Rogers and Valerie Mandelson.

Kohner N, Leftwich A. *Pregnancy Loss and the Death of a Baby* (training pack). London: National Extension College; 1995.
Supports updated SANDS guidelines for professionals.

Machin L. *Working with Young People in Loss Situations*. London: Longman; 1993.
Offers practical material, including picture triggers and worksheets that can be photocopied for direct work with children.

TEACHERNET
Website developed by the Department for Children, Schools and Families, containing lesson plans and PSHE resources. www.teachernet.gov.uk/healthandsafety

Ward B, and Associates. *Good Grief: exploring feelings, loss and death. Vol. 1: Under 11s. Vol. 2: Over 11s and adults*. London: Jessica Kingsley; 1992.
A curriculum pack of varied resources for both teachers and students.

Winston's Wish
Produces a range of activity sheets for working with grieving children, and useful guidelines for teachers in responding to a school-related death.

See Appendix A for contact details.

Videos

On the Death of a Child: a portrait of family grief (named after this book) 20 mins
Addresses different aspects of family grief, with anecdotes and commentary. Accompanying learning pack includes useful discussion points and references.
Produced by ACORNS Children's Hospice Trust, Education & Training Unit, Drakes Court, 302 Alcester Road, Wythall B47 6JR
01564 825000   www.acorns.org.uk

That Morning I Went to School 12 mins
Shows children of different ages talking about their own experiences of bereavement, their reactions and needs.
Available from Social Work Dept, Northampton General Hospital, Northampton NN1 5BD.

Giving Sorrow Words 37 mins
Useful for school staff training or individual teachers. Deals with breaking the news of a death and helping children return to school after bereavement.
Available from Video Inset, PO Box 197, Cardiff CF5 2WF

It Will Be OK 15 mins
Features young people aged 13 to 18 talking about bereavement and grief.

A Death in the Lives of . . . 18 mins
A group of 13–16 year olds talk about their experiences.
Both available from National Children's Bureau, 8 Wakley Street, London
  EC1V 7QE 020 7843 6309   www.childhoodbereavementnetwork.org.
  uk

Grief in the Family 14 mins (2002)
Animated video narrated by Michael Rosen, for families dealing with
  bereavement.

Not Too Young to Grieve 14 mins (2005)
Animated video narrated by Alison Steadman, for carers dealing with
  bereavement in under-fives.

Teenage Grief 13 mins (2007)
Animated video narrated by Lenny Henry, for those supporting bereaved
  teenagers.
These three available from: www.leedsanimation.org.uk

Don't Die of Embarrassment 18 mins (2007)
Deals with issues leading to a boy taking his own life – devised and acted
  by secondary pupils.
Produced by Papyrus www.papyrus-uk.org

Games
Board game *All About Me* produced by Peta Hemmings and available from
  Barnados.
Useful resource for adults working with primary age children.

The Grief Game produced by Yvonne Searle and Isabelle Streng, published
  by Jessica Kingsley.

Books for adults supporting children
Brown E. *Loss, Change and Grief: an educational perspective.* London: David
  Fulton; 1999.

Buckman R. *How to Break Bad News: a guide for healthcare professionals.*
  London: Papermac; 1992.

Cathcart F. *Understanding Death and Dying*. Kidderminster: British Institute of Learning Disabilities; 1994.
A booklet for carers, families, professionals.

Downey A. *Dear Stephen*. London: Arthur James; 1990.
About the suicide of a son.

Dwivedi KN, editor. *Groupwork with Children and Adolescents: a handbook*. London: Jessica Kingsley; 1993.

Dyregrov A. *Grief in Children: a handbook for adults*. London: Jessica Kingsley; 1991.

Fabian A. *The Daniel Diary*. London: Grafton Books; 1988.
Shows how young children mourn.

Fitzgerald H. *The Grieving Child: a patient's guide*. London: Simon and Schuster; 1992.

Grollman EA. *Talking About Death*. Boston: Beacon; 1990.

Jewett C. *Helping Children Cope with Separation and Loss*. London: Batsford; 1984.

Johnson J. *Suicide of a Child*. Omaha: Centering Corporation; 1984.

Leaman O. *Death and Loss: compassionate approaches in the classroom*. London: Cassell; 1995.

Lendrum S, Syme G. *Gift of Tears*. Routledge, London; 1992.

Mallon B. *Helping Children to Manage Loss*. London: Jessica Kingsley; 1998.

Mallon B. *Managing Loss, Separation and Bereavement: best policy and practice*. Manchester: Education Matters; 2000.

Pennells M, Smith S, editors. *Interventions with Bereaved Children*. London: Jessica Kingsley; 1995.

Pincus L. *Death and the Family*. London: Faber & Faber; 1976.

Shawe M, editor. *Enduring, Sharing, Loving*. London: Darton, Longman & Todd; 1992.

Silverman P. *Never Too Young to Know: death in children's lives*. Oxford: Oxford University Press; 1999.

Smith S. *The Forgotten Mourners: guidelines for working with bereaved children.* 2nd ed. London: Jessica Kingsley; 1999.

Turner M. *Talking with Children and Young People about Death and Dying: a workbook.* London: Jessica Kingsley; 1998.

Wells R. *Helping Children Cope with Grief.* London: Sheldon Press; 1988.

Wilkinson T. *The Death of a Child: a book for families.* London: Julia MacRae Books; 1991.

Winston's Wish. *Supporting a Child who is Bereaved through Suicide.* Available at www.winstonswish.org.uk (accessed 29 June 2009).

Books for younger children

Brown LK, Brown M. *When Dinosaurs Die: a guide to understanding death.* Boston: Little Brown & Co; 1996.
A multicultural look at dying and surrounding customs.

Buscaglia L. *The Fall of Freddie The Leaf.* Thorofare, NJ: Charles Slack; 1982.
Life and death allegory.

Cohn J. *I Had a Friend Named Peter: talking to children about the death of a friend.* New York: William Morrow & Co; 1987.
Betsy's friend is killed by a car.

Fitzgerald H. *The Grieving Teen.* New York: Simon & Schuster; 2000.

Fitzgerald S. *The Tale of Two Dolphins (when my sister died suddenly).* Worcs: Brambles Press; 1998.

Harper A. *Remembering Michael.* London: SANDS; 1994.
Baby brother dies at birth.

Heegaard M. *When Someone Very Special Dies.* Minneapolis: Woodland Press, 1991.
For children to illustrate their own story and feelings.

Johnson J. *Where's Jess?* Omaha: Centering Corporation; 1985.
Death of four-year-old's sibling.

Maple M. *On the Wings of a Butterfly.* Seattle: Parenting Press; 1992.
Story about a girl coping with cancer.

Nystrom C. *What Happens When We Die?* Chicago, IL: Moody Press; 1981.

Rosen M, Blake Q. *Michael Rosen's Sad Book.* London: Walker Books; 2008.

Smith HI. *When Your Friend Dies.* Minneapolis: Augsburg Fortress Publishers; 2000.

Stickney D. *Waterbugs and Dragonflies.* London: Mowbray; 1982.
An image for life and death.

Varley S. *Badger's Parting Gifts.* London: Hodder & Stoughton; 1985.
Remembering a loved friend.

Viorst J. *The Tenth Good Thing About Barney.* New York: Athenaeum; 1971.
How a young boy copes with death of a cat.

Williams M. *The Velveteen Rabbit.* New York: Avon Books; 1975.

Wilson J. *The Cat Mummy.* London: Corgi; 2002.

Books for older children
Grollman EA. *Bereaved Children and Teens.* Boston, MA: Beacon Press; 1995.

Grollman EA. *Straight Talk about Death for Teenagers: how to cope with losing someone you love.* Boston, MA: Beacon Press; 1993.

Grollman S. *Shira: a legacy of courage.* New York: Doubleday; 1988.
Coming to terms with own death and others' reactions.

Hill D. *See Ya Simon.* London: Puffin; 1995.
A teenager's last year with a dying friend.

Hipp E. *Help for the Hard Times: getting through loss.* Minnesota: Hazelden; 1995.
Self-help workbook.

Hoffman A. *At Risk.* New York: GP Putnam's Sons; 1988.
Story of 11-year-old girl with AIDS.

Kuklin S. *After a Suicide: young people speak up.* New York: GP Putnam's Sons; 1994.
Teenagers dealing with suicide of others, including friends.

Lowry L. *A Summer to Die.* Machesney Park, IL: Skylark; 1993.
Death of 13-year-old girl's older sister from leukaemia.

Richter E. *Losing Someone You Love*. New York: GP Putnam's Sons; 1986.
Young people share experiences about death of a sibling.

Vogel IM. *My Twin Sister, Erika*. New York: Harper and Row; 1986.
Loss of twin sister.

Windsor P. *The Summer Before*. New York: Harper and Row; 1973.
Girl's journal about boyfriend's accidental death.

Books for learning-disabled children

Cathcart F. *Understanding Death and Dying*. Kidderminster: British Institute
of Learning Disability; 1994.

Morris L, Perkins G. *Remembering My Brother*. London: A & C Black; 1996.

The books listed above are only a small proportion of the vast number of
books now available. The rationale for my selection is simply that I prefer
to recommend books that I know. For some more detailed book lists, try
the following websites:

www.chums.info/books

www.mariecurie.org.uk

www.winstonswish.org.uk

www.fsid.org.uk

Use of geneograms in bereavement counselling

WHAT IS A GENEOGRAM AND WHAT ARE ITS USES?

A geneogram, or genogram, is a diagrammatic representation of a family. Constructing a geneogram with a client has many possible uses:

➤ 'getting to know you'
➤ as a means of valuing and paying good attention to the client
➤ sorting out who's who in the family
➤ gaining awareness of significant relationships
➤ gaining awareness of significant dates and ages
➤ gaining awareness of significant deaths and other losses
➤ gaining awareness of significant generational and cultural patterns
➤ enabling the client to see their story from a different perspective
➤ sharing information with others (with the client's permission), for example in supervision.

In bereavement counselling the obvious benefit of a geneogram is being able to consider the deaths and losses that have affected the individual in the context of family structures and relationships. Otherwise, it is all too easy for the counsellor to assume, or to miss, the significance of any particular loss. As in the case of Louise in the example given below, contextual events may either exacerbate a bereavement or they may disguise the extent of the loss experienced. The overall picture provided by a geneogram also makes apparent the client's support structure, or lack of it. The counsellor can also discover what the client has learned from dealing with previous losses to help deal with the current loss. Making a neat copy for the client from the rough draft completed in the session can prove a useful aid to developing the 'internal supervisor' – that part of a practitioner's awareness which is self-monitoring.

This is all helpful to both the client and the counsellor, but the greatest benefit of constructing a geneogram may be to the client. There is something powerful about seeing one's place in the family objectively, and perhaps seeing it all plotted on paper may give the client permission to appreciate the extent of their losses for the first time. I remember well the impact on a client of mine who was faced with the reality of being raised by her grandmother as her own child. This proved a challenge for me, in lining her up with half-siblings previously considered as nephews and nieces, and placing her 'sister' in the generation above her as her biological mother! But for the client, her challenge came with the first real understanding of what she already knew at some level but had never allowed herself to know at another. This presented the opportunity of knowing her proper place in the family and the chance to grieve her 'mum' in a way which made space for acknowledging her real mother.

The construction of a geneogram, perhaps at a first meeting, may sound mechanistic, but in practice it offers a non-threatening and collegiate approach to the work in hand. Sitting side-by-side to sketch out a draft of the client's family story demonstrates a respectful and interested attitude. I have found it also helps the client to feel more in control of how she tells her story without becoming totally overwhelmed by her feelings. How much to prompt and ask without being intrusive or directive is something that comes with practice. In fact, an interested reader is well advised to practise this technique on willing family members and friends, and to ask a colleague to help the reader with constructing their own geneogram to see what it feels like.

How to construct a geneogram

While there are many variations in format, the basic structure to represent blood relations and other relationships is the same. Some practitioners prefer to put together a geneogram from the client's oral history without involving the client, but as stated above there are benefits from doing this together. It is essential either way to have the client's permission.

A note of caution: Geneograms follow a traditional structure of 'family' which may not easily accommodate modern patterns and alternative lifestyles. Take care that your approach gives equal value to difference. Do not, for example, assume that a partner is the opposite gender, or that children share the same parents.

The following guidelines are basic:

➤ use a different symbol for male and female (*see* example below)
➤ keep the same generation on the same level
➤ unbroken line between symbols denotes a marriage or civil partnership
➤ broken horizontal line between symbols denotes other partnerships or intimate relationships
➤ horizontal lines *above* symbols link siblings – twins have a double line
➤ vertical lines connect different generations
➤ a shaded or crossed symbol denotes death
➤ important dates and places can be written above lines and symbols, and other information may be placed underneath symbols (such as a significant feature or word to describe someone)
➤ a dash across a horizontal line denotes separation, with a double dash for divorce
➤ include miscarriages and stillbirths
➤ include pets and significant others treated as family
➤ adjectives to describe important relationships can be written on lines drawn between symbols, perhaps using different colours.

After that, you can add your own embellishments!

Example

Louise came for counselling in February 2009. She and her husband have recently moved to a lovely house in Chester after a big promotion for Simon. They are both delighted to be expecting their second child, having lost their first child, Jake, from a cot death when eight months old. Jake's sudden death was traumatic but described as 'all behind us now'. Why then can Louise not stop crying?

This simple family diagram (*see* Figure A.1) proves revealing to the counsellor, and more importantly helps Louise herself to stand back and recognise the extent of her losses. Some of these losses have been difficult to grieve, such as the sacrifices in the move to Chester; some have been hidden, such as the termination; and some have been juxtaposed with birth or other

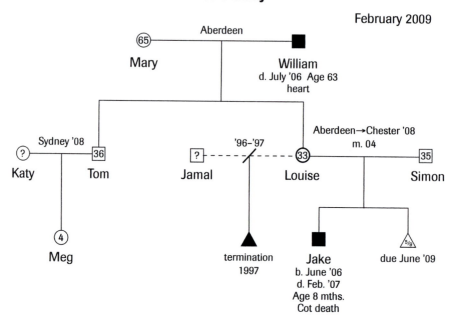

Louise's family

February 2009

celebrations, such as the death of Louise's father shortly after Jake's birth. Louise can now see how much the 'positive' move to Chester has displaced her from everything associated with Jake – including his grave – and this anniversary time has triggered another layer of grieving. She also becomes aware of how many feelings will be stirred by the timing of the arrival of the new baby, which will coincide with Jake's birthday and the anniversary of William's death.

In addition, the geneogram has clarified the disruption of her family support network, with her mother back in Aberdeen and her brother's move to Australia.

(Louise and her family are fictional.)

Reference

McGoldrick M. *Genograms: assessment and intervention.* New York: Norton Professional Books; 2008.

Essential references

Ayalon O, Flasher A. *Chain Reaction*. London: Jessica Kingsley; 1993.

Bowlby J. *Attachment and Loss*, Vols 1–3. *Attachment*, Vol. 1, 1969; *Separation: anxiety and anger*, Vol. 2, 1973; *Loss: sadness and depression*, Vol. 3, 1980. New York: Basic Books; 1969–80.

Buckman R. *How to Break Bad News: a guide for healthcare professionals*. London: Papermac; 1992.

Capewell E. Critical incident management in schools: headteachers' briefing. *Croner*. 1993; **28**: 4–5 and **29**: 5–7.

Capewell E. Responding to children in trauma: a systems approach for schools. *Bereavement Care*. 1994; **13**(1): 2–7.

Cheshire County Council. *Managing the Response to Critical Incidents in Schools*. Chester: CCC; 2007. (Now separated into Cheshire East Council and Cheshire West and Chester.)

Dent A. A study of bereavement care after a sudden and unexpected death. *Arch Dis Child*. 1996; **74**(6): 522–6.

Dyregrov A. *Grief in Children*. London: Jessica Kingsley; 1994.

Green J. *Death with Dignity: meeting the spiritual needs of patients in a multi-cultural society*. London: Macmillan Magazines; 1991.

Grollman EA. *Talking About Death: a dialogue between parent and child*. Boston: Beacon Press; 1990.

Herbert M. *Supporting Bereaved and Dying Children and Their Parents*. Leicester: The British Psychological Society; 1996.

Hill L, editor. *Caring for Dying Children and Their Families*. London: Chapman & Hall; 1994.

Hindmarch C. Secondary losses for siblings. *Child Care Health Dev*. 1995; **21**(6): 425–31.

Joseph S, Linley PA. *Positive Therapy. A meta-theory for positive psychological practice*. London: Routledge; 2006.

Joseph S, Linley P. Positive adjustment to threatening events: an organismic valuing theory of growth through adversity. *Rev Gen Psychol.* 2005; 9: 455–71.

Klass D. *The Spiritual Lives of Bereaved Parents.* Philadelphia: Bruner/Mazel; 1999.

Klass D, Silverman P, Nickman S, editors. *Continuing Bonds: new understandings of grief.* London: Taylor & Francis; 1996.

Lendrum S, Syme G. *Gift of Tears.* London: Routledge; 1992.

Machin L. *Working with Loss and Grief.* Thousand Oaks, CA: Sage Publications; 2009.

O'Hara DM, Taylor R, Simpson K. Critical incident stress debriefing: bereavement support in schools – Developing a role for an LA educational psychology service. *Educ Psych in Practice.* 1994; 10(1): 27–34.

Parkes CM, Relf M, Couldrick A. *Counselling in Terminal Care and Bereavement.* Baltimore: BPS Books; 1996.

Stewart J. *Guidelines for Setting Up a Bereavement Service.* London: National Association of Bereavement Services; 1991.

Stroebe M, Stroebe W, Hansson R, editors. *Handbook of Bereavement: theory, research and intervention.* Cambridge: Cambridge University Press; 1993.

Talbot K. *What Forever Means after the Death of a Child: transcending the trauma, living with loss.* New York: Brunner-Routledge; 2002.

Turner M. *Talking with Children and Young People about Death and Dying.* London: Jessica Kingsley; 1998.

Worden WJ. *Grief Counselling and Grief Therapy.* 4th ed. London: Routledge; 2008.

Yalom I. *Staring at the Sun: overcoming the dread of death.* London: Piatkus; 2008.

Yule W, Gold A. *Wise Before the Event: coping with crises in schools.* London: Gulbenkian Foundation; 1993.

Further reading

There is such a wide range of books and articles written about children and death that the list of titles below cannot be comprehensive. These titles have been selected on the basis of what is known to the author personally or by recommendation.

Arnold JH, Buschman Gemma P. *A Child Dies*. 2nd ed. Philadelphia: The Charles Press; 1994.

Balk D. The self-concept of bereaved adolescents: sibling death and its aftermath. *J Adolesc Res*. 1990; **5**(1): 112–32.

Barnard P, Morland I, Nagy J. *Children, Bereavement and Trauma: nurturing resilience*. London: Jessica Kingsley; 1999.

Bertman SL. *Facing Death: images, insights and interventions*. New York: Hemisphere Publishing Corporation; 1991.

Birenbaum LK, Robinson MA, Phillips DS, Stewart BJ. The response of children to the dying and death of a sibling. *Omega*. 1989–90; **20**(3): 213–28.

Black D, Urbanowicz MA. Family intervention with bereaved children. *J Child Psychol Psychiatry*. 1987; **28**: 467–76.

Bluebond-Langner M. *The Private Worlds of Dying Children*. Princeton: Princeton University Press; 1978.

Bluebond-Langner M. *Worlds of dying children and their well siblings*. In: Doka K, editor. *Children Mourning, Mourning Children*. Washington, DC: Hospice Association of America; 1995.

Bowlby J. *The Making and Breaking of Affectionate Bonds*. London: Tavistock; 1979.

Brooks B, Siegel P. *The Scared Child: helping kids overcome traumatic events*. Chichester: John Wiley & Sons; 1996.

Brown E. *Loss, Change and Grief: an educational perspective*. London: David Fulton Publishers; 1999.

Buckman R. *I Don't Know What to Say: how to help and support someone who is dying.* London: Papermac; 1988.

Capewell E. *Systems for Managing Crisis Incidents in Schools.* London: Capewell; 1994.

Cook B, Phillips S. *Loss and Bereavement.* London: Austen Cornish: 1988.

Couldrick A. *Grief and Bereavement: understanding children.* Oxford: Sobell Publications; 1991.

Dickinson D, Johnson M, editors. *Death, Dying and Bereavement.* London: Sage Publications; 1993.

Doka K, editor. *Children Mourning, Mourning Children.* Washington, DC: Hospice Association of America; 1995.

Donnelly KF. *Recovering From the Loss of a Sibling.* New York: Dodd Mead; 1988.

Duffy W. *Children and Bereavement.* London: National Society/Church House Publishing; 1995.

Dwivedi KN, editor. *Groupwork with Children and Adolescents: a handbook.* London: Jessica Kingsley; 1993.

Dyregrov A, Mathieson S. Anxiety and vulnerability in parents following the death of an infant. *Scand J Psychol.* 1987; **28**: 16–25.

Farrant A. *Sibling Bereavement: helping children cope with loss.* London: Cassell; 1998.

Finkbeiner AK. *After the Death of a Child: living in Loss.* Baltimore: Johns Hopkins University Press; 1996.

Finlay I, Dallimore D. Your child is dead. *BMJ.* 1991; **302**: 1524–5.

Gatliffe ED. *Death in the Classroom: a resource book for teachers and others.* London: Epworth Press; 1988.

Gullo S. *Death and Children.* New York: Dobbs Ferry; 1985.

Hawkins P, Shohet R. *Supervision in the Helping Professions.* 3rd ed. Buckingham: Open University Press; 2007.

Hawton K. *Suicide and Attempted Suicide Among Children.* London: Sage Publications; 1986.

Herbert M. *PTSD in Children.* London: BPS Books; 1996.

Hodgkinson P, Stewart M. *Coping with Catastrophe: a handbook of disaster management.* London: Routledge; 1991.

Hogan N, Greenfield D. Adolescent sibling bereavement. *J Adolesc Res.* 1991; **6**(1): 108.

Hornby G. *Working with Parents of Children with Special Needs.* London: Cassell; 1995.

James IA. Helping people with learning difficulties to cope with bereavement. *Br J Learn Disabil.* 1995; **23**: 74–8.

Jewett C. *Helping Children Cope With Separation and Loss.* London: Batsford; 1984.

Johnson J. *Suicide of a Child.* Omaha: Centering Corporation; 1984.

Judd D. *Give Sorrow Words: working with a dying child*. London: Free Association Books; 1990.

Kinchin D. *Post Traumatic Stress Disorder: the invisible injury*. Wantage: Success Unlimited; 1998.

Klass D. The deceased child in the psychic and social worlds of bereaved parents during the resolution of grief. *Death Stud.* 1997; **21**(2): 147–75.

Knapp RJ. *Beyond Endurance: when a child dies*. New York: Schocken; 1986.

Knight B. *Sudden Death in Infancy*. London: Faber & Faber; 1983.

Kohner N, Henley A. *When a Baby Dies*. London: Stillbirth and Neonatal Death Society; 1991.

Kubler-Ross E. *On Death and Dying*. London: Tavistock Press; 1970.

Kubler-Ross E. *On Children and Death*. London: Macmillan; 1983.

Lamberti J. Model of family grief assessment and treatment. *Death Stud.* 1993; **17**: 55–67.

Lang A, Gottlieb L. Parental grief reactions and marital intimacy following infant death. *Death Stud.* 1993; **17**: 233–55.

Leaman O. *Death and Loss: compassionate approaches in the classroom*. London: Cassell; 1995.

Littlewood J. *Aspects of Grief*. London: Routledge; 1992.

Mallon B. *Helping Children to Manage Loss*. London: Jessica Kingsley; 1998.

McCollum A. *The Chronically Ill Child: a guide for parents and professionals*. New Haven: Yale University Press; 1975.

Mearns D, Thorne B. *Person-Centred Counselling in Action*. London: Sage Publications; 1988.

Miller S, Ober D. *Finding Hope When a Child Dies: what other cultures can teach us*. New York: Fireside Books; 2002.

Moddia B. Grief reactions and learning disabilities. *Nurs Stand.* 1992; **9**(33): 38–9.

Oakley A, McPherson A, Roberts H. *Miscarriage*. London: Fontana; 1984.

Parkes CM, Relf M, Couldrick A. *Counselling in Terminal Care and Bereavement*. London: British Psychological Society; 1996.

Parkes CM. Weiss RS. *Recovery from Bereavement*. New York: Basic Books; 1983.

Pennells M, Smith S. *The Forgotten Mourners: guidelines for working with bereaved children*. London: Jessica Kingsley; 1995.

Pettle MSA, Lansdown RG. Adjustment to death of a sibling. *Arch Dis Child.* 1986; **61**: 278–83.

Pincus L. *Death and the Family*. London: Faber & Faber; 1976.

Rando TA. An investigation of grief and adaptation in parents whose children have died from cancer. *J Pediatr Psychol.* 1983; **8**: 3–20.

Rando TA. *Parental Loss of a Child*. Champaign: Research Press; 1986.

Raphael B. *The Anatomy of Bereavement: a handbook for the caring professions*. London: Unwin Hyman; 1984.

Raphael B. *When Disaster Strikes: a handbook for the caring professions*. London: Unwin Hayman; 1986.

Sanders CM. A comparison of adult bereavement in the death of a spouse, child and parent. *Omega*. 1979–80; **10**(4): 303–23.

Sanders P. *A Complete Guide to Using Counselling Skills on the Telephone*. Manchester: PCCS Books; 1993.

Scott MJ, Palmer S, editors. *Trauma and Post-traumatic Stress Disorder*. London: Cassell; 2000.

Segal R. Helping children express grief through symbolic communication. *Soc Casework: J Contemp Soc Work*. 1984; **65**(6): 590–9.

Shawe M, editor. *Enduring, Sharing, Loving*. London: Darton, Longman & Todd; 1992.

Smith S, Pennells M. *Interventions with Bereaved Children*. London: Jessica Kingsley; 1995.

Speck P. *Loss and Grief in Medicine*. London: Bailliere Tindall; 1978.

Spinetta JJ. The dying child's awareness of death: a review. *Psychol Bull*. 1974; **81**: 841–5.

Staudacher C. *Beyond Grief*. London: Souvenir Press; 1988.

Staudacher C. *Men and Grief*. London: Souvenir Press; 1991.

Stedeford A. *Facing Death: patients, families and professionals*. Oxford: Heinemann; 1984.

Tatelbaum J. *The Courage to Grieve*. Oxford: Heinemann; 1981.

Taylor Warmbrod M. Counselling bereaved children: stages in the process. *Soc Casework: J Contemp Soc Work*. 1986; **67**(6): 351–8.

Vachon M. *Occupational Stress in the Care of the Critically Ill, the Dying and the Bereaved*. Washington, DC: Hemisphere; 1981.

Walter T. A new model of grief bereavement and biography. *Mortality*. 1996; **1**(1): 7–25.

Ward B and Associates. *Good Grief: exploring feelings, loss and death (Vol. 1: Under 11s. Vol. 2: Over 11s and adults)*. 2nd ed. London: Jessica Kingsley; 1993.

Wells R. *Helping Children Cope with Grief*. London: Sheldon Press; 1988.

Wilkinson T. *The Death of a Child: a book for families*. London: Julia MacRae Books; 1991.

Zaiger N. Women and bereavement. *Women Ther*. 1986; **4**: 1985–6.

Index